"The authors have taken a vast range of relevant material and delivered an enlightening and provocative resource for students and others dealing with the complexities of child welfare today."

—*Daniel Pollack, Professor, Wurzweiler School of Social Work, Yeshiva University*

"Child Welfare: Preparing Social Workers for Practice in the Field is a comprehensive and practical blending of theory, practice, and policy in this critical arena of social work. The authors use multiple case examples and describe pertinent court decisions to explain the evolution and challenges of child welfare services. The examples bring cases to life and worksheets and drawings illustrate the kinds of tasks with which social workers must deal. I was particularly impressed with the discussion about mandated reporting, assessment using the person-in-environment model, and the difficulties of youth aging out of foster care. I believe that the book represents a solid addition to the knowledge base of social work and that students will find it compelling reading."

—*Grafton H. Hull Jr., Professor Emeritus at the University of Utah College of Social Work*

Child Welfare

Child Welfare: Preparing Social Workers for Practice in the Field is a comprehensive text for child welfare courses taught from a social work perspective. This textbook provides a single source for all material necessary for a contextual child welfare course.

As well as combining history, theory, and practice, the authors integrate different practice perspectives to teach social workers how to engage children and families at the micro, mezzo, and macro levels. Covering both broad issues, such as child welfare, child maltreatment, and responses to child maltreatment, and current issues in social care, including mandated reporting and evidence-based policy prevention and preservation, the material is designed to meet the needs of social work students entering the child welfare workforce.

Child Welfare provides students in social work courses at both the undergraduate and graduate levels with a single source for all material necessary to successfully navigate their studies and careers.

Kathryn Krase, Associate Professor of Social Work in the Wurzweiler School of Social Work at Yeshiva University, is an expert in the Mandated Reporting of Suspected Child Maltreatment, with many significant publications and presentations on the topic. As a lawyer, Dr. Krase represented children in Family Court for the New York Society for the Prevention of Cruelty to Children.

Tobi DeLong Hamilton, Assistant Professor and MSW Program Director in the Department of Social Work at Brandman University, has worked in the social work field for 20 years and has experience in child welfare, adoptions, medical and psychiatric social work. She worked in private practice as a psychotherapist specializing in family and childhood problems prior to moving into higher education full time. While in private practice, she maintained a connection to public child welfare by evaluating, writing reports, and testifying as an expert witness for children in foster care.

Child Welfare

Preparing Social Workers for Practice in the Field

**Kathryn Krase and
Tobi DeLong Hamilton**

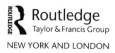
Routledge
Taylor & Francis Group

NEW YORK AND LONDON

First published 2021
by Routledge
52 Vanderbilt Avenue, New York, NY 10017

and by Routledge
2 Park Square, Milton Park, Abingdon, Oxon OX14 4RN

Routledge is an imprint of the Taylor & Francis Group, an informa business

© 2021 Taylor & Francis

The right of Kathryn Krase and Tobi DeLong Hamilton to be identified as authors of this work has been asserted by them in accordance with sections 77 and 78 of the Copyright, Designs and Patents Act 1988.

Library of Congress Cataloging-in-Publication Data
Names: Krase, Kathryn, author. | DeLong Hamilton, Tobi, author.
Title: Child welfare : preparing social workers for practice in the field / Kathryn Krase, Tobi DeLong Hamilton.
Description: 1 Edition. | New York City : Routledge Books, 2020. | Includes bibliographical references and index.
Identifiers: LCCN 2020029012 | ISBN 9781138218826 (hardback) | ISBN 9781138218833 (paperback) | ISBN 9781315437019 (ebook)
Subjects: LCSH: Child welfare. | Social work with children.
Classification: LCC HV713 .K73 2020 | DDC 362.7–dc23
LC record available at https://lccn.loc.gov/2020029012

ISBN: 978-1-138-21882-6 (hbk)
ISBN: 978-1-138-21883-3 (pbk)
ISBN: 978-1-315-43701-9 (ebk)

Typeset in Bembo
by Taylor & Francis Books

Contents

Illustrations

Figures

Tables

Part I

A Social Work Introduction to Child Welfare

1   What Is Child Welfare?

Chapter Summary

In order to understand the policies and systems designed to protect children from harm, we need to understand the basic concepts that frame "Child Welfare". Who is a child? What do children need? What is "welfare"? Who is responsible for preserving child welfare? These may seem like straight-forward questions, with simple answers, but this chapter will, hopefully, make clear that there are no simple answers, because these questions are more complex than first imagined.

Defining Child Welfare

In the field of social work, when someone mentions "child welfare" they are usually referring to a large system made up of governmental and private entities who have a level of responsibility for protecting children from harm at the hands of their families or caretakers. The term "child welfare system" generally includes child protective services, governmental and privately operated systems that coordinate out-of-home placement of children, and other related services provided by the government or non-governmental agencies. The child welfare system is designed to protect children from certain types of harm. To better understand how this system works, it is important to understand the underlying concepts that define it.

Who Is a Child?

The question, Who is a child? has a simple answer in the United States: anyone under 18 years of age. Children are not allowed to make many decisions for themselves. For instance, parents, not children, get to decide what school children go to, what medicine children take when sick, how much screen time children can have on a daily basis, and what YouTube channels children can access. From a legal perspective, children cannot make most decisions about their own care and well-being. For instance, a child, generally, needs a parent or other legal guardian to provide authorization for most medical procedures or permission to even go on a school trip.

In all states, when a competent person attains their 18th birthday, they gain certain legal rights that allow them to make a plethora of decisions for themselves. Turning 18 is often referred to as "reaching majority". This is why individuals under 18 years old are often referred to as "minors". At 18 years of age, an individual can enter into a legal contract. At 18, an individual can get married in any state without parental permission. At 18, an individual can enlist in the armed forces without parental permission. While many young adults may still reside with their parents, having reached adulthood, their parents are no longer responsible for providing or caring for them.

There are, however, many people who are 18 years of age, or older, who continue to have limited rights. When someone with a physical, mental, or cognitive impairment is determined by a court to be unable to make competent decisions to preserve their own well-being, another adult, or the government, will be assigned as "guardian" and held responsible for making such decisions. In many states, the same systems put in place to protect "child welfare" will serve to protect the welfare of incompetent/incapacitated adults.

Additionally, individuals who were in out-of-home placement prior to turning 18 are often allowed to remain in the child welfare system after they attain majority. These individuals have all the legal rights of adults, but the government retains some responsibility for caring for them until they reach a certain age (depending on the state), or they transition out of the child welfare system.

The larger question here is, Why does society define the term "child"? The answer to that question is more complex. The next chapter presents an historical analysis of child welfare that gets into detail about changing societal understanding of who a child is. At the most basic level, though, we define the term child so that we, as a society, can respond differently to the rights and responsibilities related to the group. While 18 as the age of majority is roughly related to developmental expectations for maturity and the ability to care for oneself, in reality 18 is an arbitrary number. Some individuals may be mature enough to take care of themselves at 16 or 17, while others may not be similarly responsible until deep into their 20s, if ever. However, it would be a governmental nightmare to determine who is a child and who is an adult on an individual basis. (You think the line at the Department of Motor Vehicles is bad ....)

For the purposes of the present discussion on the child welfare system and throughout this text, we use the general American standard to define childhood: a child is under 18 years of age unless the individual is deemed incompetent/incapacitated by the government or the individual remains under the authority of the child welfare system due to their status in out-of-home placement beyond their 18th birthday.

What Is "Welfare"

When most people hear the term "welfare" they think of governmental services provided to poor people. However, the term "welfare" is much simpler than that. "Welfare" means "the state of doing well". Therefore, "child welfare" simply refers to efforts to preserve or improve the health or condition of children.

In order to determine the welfare of a child, society has expectations for what children need. The concept of "well-being" takes into account many facets of a child's condition in an effort to determine if their needs are being met. At the most basic level, to ensure survival a child needs food, shelter, and clothing. In twenty-first-century America, however, no one thinks that basic levels are enough. Children are expected to have access to the medical system to ensure their health. Children are expected to have access to the educational system to ensure they learn the skills necessary to become independent adults. Children are also expected to be protected from harm, more so than adults are protected.

But are food, shelter, clothing, medical care, education, and safety enough? What else do we think children need? Do children need to be clean? Do children need to be physically active? Do children need adequate rest? Do children need to be happy? Does society have any structures in place that are designed to meet children's other needs? Should society develop new structures to meet other needs?

What Is Sufficient?

It is not revolutionary to say that children need basic standards of food, shelter, and clothing to support their welfare. But what are the standards? Is it enough that children are given the opportunity to eat food sufficient to meet their dietary requirements for growth, a place to sleep out of nature's elements, or clothing appropriate for the weather? Or should children be guaranteed the healthiest foods? Should children have their own bed to sleep in? Are hand-me-downs or less-than-fashionable clothes sufficient?

When considering and applying standards in child welfare, it is important to note that there are different standards for what is acceptable. Families of different socioeconomic levels or from different cultures may have different expectations for what is enough. When a social worker is in the process of evaluating whether a child is receiving adequate resources to support their welfare, it is important to be aware of any personal experiences or expectations that may impact such an assessment and, instead, use objective criteria that eliminate the impact of bias.

Who Is Responsible for Child Welfare?

Now that we have a basic understanding of who children are and what they need to support their welfare, the next question is the whole reason for this book: Whose responsibility is it to ensure that children's welfare is protected?

This used to be an easy question. Until the late nineteenth century the answer was simply: the parents. As you will see in the next chapter, those expectations have changed a lot since 1875. The answer in the present time is different. A combination of parents, other family members, the government, and even, sometimes, children are responsible for ensuring that children's welfare is protected.

Role of Children

It may seem unfair to expect children to be responsible for their own welfare. But, when you really think about it, much of childhood is spent teaching children how to be responsible for their own welfare so that they are ready when adulthood arrives.

Expectations that children preserve their own welfare vary by age or developmental stage. No one expects a toddler to make responsible food choices or know when it is time to take a nap. However, there is a point at which children can toilet themselves or adequately brush their own teeth (without supervision).

Due to evolving expectations regarding children's responsibility for their own welfare, the standards expected of their caretakers differ depending on the child's age and developmental stage. For instance, when a 7-year-old is not attending school regularly, the parents may likely be found responsible for educational neglect. However, when a 15-year-old is not attending school regularly, the child welfare system is more likely to consider the teenager's role in failing to meet the educational standard. It is important to note that, even when a child is determined to have contributed to a condition contrary to promotion of their own welfare, their parents will ultimately be held responsible for ensuring improvement.

Role of Parents

Why do we hold parents responsible for their own children? In some cultures, children born into a community are the responsibility of all. However, in America, the expectation is that children will be cared for by their parents first. If parents fail in their responsibility, then we have mechanisms in place to fill the parental role.

Parents in the United States of America have many rights when it comes to the care of their children. Many of these rights are codified through important United States Supreme Court decisions.

Parents have the right to, largely, determine their child's education. In the 1923 case of *Meyer v. Nebraska* (262 U.S. 390), an instructor at a parochial school was tried and convicted of a crime for teaching children in a foreign language (German). Nebraska had a criminal statute, the Siman Act, that outlawed the teaching in foreign languages to children until ninth grade in any school in the state. The law was a xenophobic response to World War I and growing immigration from Germany and Italy, much like the "English-Only" laws that were passed in Iowa and Ohio around the same time. The teacher, Robert Meyer, appealed his conviction all the way to the United States Supreme Court. In a blistering opinion, the Court struck down the Siman Act, and other acts, by a 7–2 vote. The Meyer decision was the first in a series of important Supreme Court decisions that found rights in the US Constitution that were not explicitly written in the document. In the Meyer decision, the Court determined, for the first time, that individuals have "certain fundamental rights which must be respected", including "the right to marry, establish a home, and bring up children". Included in the right to bring up children, the Court found "the power of parents to control the education of their own" children.

In 1925, just two years after the Meyer decision, the US Supreme Court came down with another important case related to parents' right to determine the education of their children: *Pierce v. Society of the Sisters of the Holy Names of Jesus and Mary* (268 U.S. 510). Similar to Nebraska, Oregon passed laws aimed at limiting the influence of immigrants. The goal was to use public education as the means to promote a common American culture through the Compulsory Education Act. The primary purpose of the Act was to require children between the ages of eight and 16 years old to attend school. However, Oregon took the law one step further, requiring students to attend *public* school, with limited exceptions. Private and parochial schools challenged the law as an overextension of State power. The US Supreme Court unanimously agreed with the private and parochial schools, striking down the Oregon law as unconstitutional. Clarifying that a child is not "the mere creature of the state", the Court found that "those who nurture [the child] and direct [the child's] destiny have the right, coupled with the high duty, to recognize and prepare [the child] for additional obligations."

Nearly 50 years after *Meyer v. Nebraska*, the Supreme Court returned to the issue of parental control over education and religion in the 1972 case *Wisconsin v. Yoder* (406 U.S. 205). The compulsory education law of Wisconsin required parents to have their children educated until they turned 16. Amish and Mennonite parents argued that their children should not be required to stay in school past the eighth grade since such preparation was not necessary to live an adult life based on their religious beliefs. The US Supreme Court sided with the parents, finding that the Wisconsin's "interest in universal education" needs to be balanced against the "fundamental rights" of parents, including the "interest of parents with respect to the religious upbringing of their children". Essentially, the Court said that the government's concerns for educating all children in the state do not outweigh the parents' right to choose to educate their children in accordance with their religious practices.

The US Supreme Court has very rarely taken up cases related to child maltreatment, foster care, or adoption since they are issues generally under the jurisdiction of states, not the federal government. However, in the 1982 case of *Santosky v. Kramer* (466 U.S. 745), the Court stepped in to set a national standard for the burden of proof required for the government to terminate parental rights.

Child maltreatment cases are handled in civil courts, not criminal courts. The burden of proof required to make a conviction in criminal court is a very high standard: "beyond a reasonable doubt". "Beyond a reasonable doubt" means that a conviction must be made only when there is no doubt, or no "reasonable" doubt, that the alleged perpetrator committed the crime. The burden of proof required to make a finding in most civil courts is much lower: "fair preponderance of the evidence". "Fair preponderance of the evidence" means that a finding must be made only when the evidence for a finding outweighs the evidence against a finding. The standard rests on the balance between two questions: Is there more evidence that supports a finding, or more evidence against? At the time of the Santosky case, in most states the burden of proof for cases in which the government sought to terminate parental rights was "fair preponderance of the evidence".

In the early 1980s, parents in New York State challenged the standard, arguing that parental rights were too valuable to be terminated under such a low standard. The US Supreme Court agreed with the parents. The Court determined that in termination of parental rights cases, the individual interests at stake (those of parental rights) were both "particularly important" and "more substantial than mere loss of money"; therefore, a higher standard, "clear and convincing evidence", should be used. The Court noted that "[when] a State initiates a parental rights termination proceeding, it seeks not merely to infringe [upon a] fundamental liberty interest, but to end it". As such, the Court determined that a higher burden of proof was called for. It is important to note that "clear and convincing evidence" is not as high a burden of proof as "beyond a reasonable doubt".

With the recognition of parental rights, there also comes the recognition of many responsibilities for parents. As the court decisions outlined above established parents' rights to make certain decisions about the upbringing of their children, societal expectations began to shift. As parents gained de facto rights, they were also held to higher standards. Failure to provide "custody, care, and nurture" or adequate education or medical care, for example, are all common cases in the child welfare system of the twenty-first century.

Role of Family

In many cultures, family members other than parents—grandparents, siblings, aunts, uncles, cousins, etc.—are expected to be responsible for the welfare of children in their family. Responsibility does not sit solely with parents. In the United States, parents have primacy in the right to determine the upbringing of their children, and non-parental family members have limited rights.

Troxel v. Granville (530 U.S. 57), an important 2000 US Supreme Court case, made clear the rights of family members other than parents. Tommie Granville and Brad Troxel had two daughters together. Their relationship ended in 1991. For the next two years, Brad cared for his daughters on the weekends. On these weekends, Brad's parents, Jenifer and Gary Troxel, were often with them. After Brad committed suicide in 1993, Tommie only allowed the grandparents to visit with the girls for a short period each month. The Troxels sued for the right to more visitation with their grand-daughters. There were no allegations that visits with the grandparents were injurious to the girls. There were no suspicions that Tommie was a bad mom either. The US Supreme Court sided with Tommie. Citing prior decisions, like *Meyer v. Nebraska* (1923), *Pierce v. Society of the Sisters of the Holy Names of Jesus and Mary* (1925), and *Wisconsin v. Yoder* (1972), the Court flatly declared that the US Constitution "protects the fundamental right of parents to make decisions concerning the care, custody, and control of their children." Since there was no concern that Tommie Granville was anything other than a competent parent, the Court said that no one had the right to question her right to determine who her children spent time with.

The *Troxel v. Granville* (2000) decision was a major blow to proponents of the rights of family members, but it solidified parents' rights under the law.

Role of Government

As you will learn in Chapter 2, the government of the United States and individual states have long histories of avoiding involvement in family matters. As a result, for much of the nation's history, the government did not assert any responsibility for ensuring the welfare of children. However, today the government is largely steeped in preserving child welfare. Because it provides public education and health insurance to tens of millions of American children, the American government currently asserts great responsibility for ensuring that children's welfare is protected. One particular 1944 US Supreme Court decision, *Prince v. Massachusetts* (321 U.S. 158), was integral to the development of these current systems.

Sarah Prince, a Jehovah's Witness, brought along her 9-year-old niece and ward, Betty Simmons, to preach on the streets of Brockton, Massachusetts. While preaching they distributed literature, *The Watchtower*, in exchange for voluntary monetary contributions. Sarah was arrested and convicted for violating child labor laws. The child labor laws at the time stipulated that no boys under 12 and no girls under 18 were permitted to sell literature or other goods on the streets. Sarah appealed her conviction, arguing that her and Betty's First Amendment rights to the free exercise of religion were violated by the child labor laws. The US Supreme Court disagreed. The Court found that the "family itself is not beyond regulation" when the government has an interest, even if there is a conflict with the First Amendment right to practice religion. The Court asserted that "neither the rights of religion nor the rights of parenthood are beyond limitation". Through the *Prince v. Massachusetts* (1944) decision the Court declared that parental authority is not absolute. Therefore, the government can restrict the rights of parents as long as the government is legitimately protecting the interests of a child's welfare.

The present United States child welfare system developed through the *Prince v. Massachusetts* (1944) decision, the other cases discussed above, and the many more that we did not discuss here. The following chapters will provide you with more context and information to guide you as you explore the role of social work in this complex area of practice.

Case Examples and Questions

1   As discussed above, the age of 18 is set as the threshold for adulthood. Using the knowledge you have gained through your studies in social work, how do you think the government should define the threshold for adulthood?

2   In 2018, contrary to past practices, the United States government separated children from their parents as they crossed the border from Mexico, creating a humanitarian crisis and causing widespread outrage. Using the concepts you learned in this chapter, including the definitions of "child" and "welfare" and the rights and responsibilities of children, parents, family, and the government, provide a rationale for and a rationale against this policy of separation. Which rationale should prevail? Why?

Further Reading

Guggenheim, M. (2005). *What's Wrong with Children's Rights?* Cambridge, MA: Harvard University Press.

References

Meyer v. Nebraska, 262 U.S. 390 (1923).
Pierce v. Society of the Sisters of the Holy Names of Jesus and Mary, 268 U.S. 510 (1925).
Prince v. Massachusetts, 321 U.S. 158 (1944).
Santosky v. Kramer, 466 U.S. 745 (1982).
Troxel v. Granville, 530 U.S. 57 (2000).
Wisconsin v. Yoder, 406 U.S. 205 (1972).

2 History of Child Welfare

Exploring How Children Have Been Treated Across History

When exploring the history of childhood, there are generally three time periods, which are defined by the prevailing theories and beliefs of the time: Indifference to Childhood (before the fifteenth century), Discovery of Childhood (fifteenth to eighteenth centuries), and Preoccupation with Childhood (nineteenth century to the present) (Empey et al., 1999).

Indifference to Childhood (Before the Fifteenth Century)

For the longest time, children were not viewed as a special population of people requiring distinct treatment or protection. Instead, children were often viewed as requiring less protection or respect since they were not considered fully formed people. As a result, parents, namely fathers, were ultimately responsible for making decisions about the care of children.

In ancient Greece (approximately 800–500 BC), children were the absolute property of their fathers. As such, fathers could do with their children as they pleased. The law allowed fathers to determine, by the child's fifth day after birth, whether the child should live. If a father did not want a child, perhaps due to family poverty, birth defect, or merely because the child was female (and, therefore, less valuable), he could cast the child out of the house to die of exposure to the elements or throw the newborn over a cliff.

In ancient Rome (approximately 600 BC–500 AD), fathers also held the power of life or death over their children into adulthood. This power was found in the legal principle of *patria potestas*, meaning "power of the father". The law ultimately developed to limit a father's powers, such that most children could not be killed before the age of three. More specifically, the law evolved to forbid the infanticide of able-bodied male children, who were deemed necessary for the development of future soldiers for the Roman Empire. If a father did not want to keep his child, the law then allowed him to sell the child into slavery instead of killing him/her.

Infanticide was increasingly looked down upon as predominant religious beliefs, on which laws and cultural practices were based, shifted from the polytheistic (multiple gods) Greek and Roman belief systems to the monotheistic (single god) orders of Judaism, Islam, and Christianity. Instead, the earliest Christian churches offered parents the opportunity to place unwanted children into the church's care.

In medieval Europe childhood was perilous. Due to poor living conditions, disease, and famine, one quarter (25%) of all children born did not live to see their first birthday. Another 25% of children did not make it to their tenth birthdays. Since the causes of these deaths were largely unpreventable, families did little to invest in children, financially or emotionally, before the likelihood of them living into adulthood was more certain. Instead, children were often considered miniature adults. They were put to work as early as possible so they could contribute to the costs of their own care.

Discovery of Childhood (Fifteenth–Eighteenth Centuries)

As infant mortality decreased in early modern England, children were more likely to live further into childhood and adulthood. Families became more willing to risk emotional attachment to children. As a result, more attention was paid to the nuances of childhood, including the way children talked and moved. A cultural appreciation for childhood experiences grew. Instead of merely treating children like small adults, children were treated differently. It is important to note, however, that the length of childhood was a lot shorter than commonly understood and appreciated today. English children of five or six years old might be considered adults, and society had the same expectations for them as for other adults. They had to work for their keep.

Residents of early American colonies were not focused on the experiences of children. Most American colonies were developed as platforms for trading the natural resources of the "New World" with Europe and beyond. As a result, the focus was largely on work. These colonies were largely populated by white men capable of strenuous physical work, male and female slaves of African descent, and a few white women, mostly in areas where slavery was not as prevalent. These white women were often relegated to tasks deemed inappropriate to white men, like cooking and cleaning. White children too young for work were often not welcome in the early colonies. Children born to slaves of African descent were often seen as commodities and as possessions of their parents' masters. Their value to white male colonists was purely economic.

Some American colonies were developed to allow the free expression of religious practices by certain communities of people who were unable to do so in the European countries of their birth, such as the Puritans of Massachusetts. These colonies had families, including women, men, and children.

White colonial children were the responsibility, morally and economically, of their parents. White colonial American children were expected "to be seen, but not heard". At mealtime they often sat at tables separate from the adults in their families. Boys as young as seven years old were matched with tradesmen as apprentices in preparation for a worthy career, or if their families had means, boys were in school. Girls were less likely to be educated or apprenticed. Instead, they took on tasks in the home in preparation for the "proper" life of women, tending to the home. White children, boys and girls, from poorer families could be sold into indentured servitude. Abandoned or orphaned children were placed in poorhouses alongside alcoholic and mentally ill adults who could not care for or financially support themselves.

Black children in early America had very different experiences compared to white children. Children born to enslaved mothers or those bought into slavery as children were the property of their masters, and their parents had no right to a relationship with them. Young enslaved children of African descent could be separated from their birth families at any time and with no input from their parents. The youngest enslaved children were usually cared for by older women and/or older children while their parents worked. Boys and girls were expected to join work as soon as they were able. Free children of African descent were the responsibility of their families. If the family was incapable of taking care of them, the children would be taken care of by the larger family network or religious community. Free children of African descent were unlikely to be served by traditional poorhouses and orphanages, which were largely restricted to serving only white people.

The discovery of childhood coincides with the beginning of social welfare policies and practices in the United States. As the Elizabethan Poor Laws of England were adopted in early American colonies, the expectation that families would meet the needs of their own, namely their children, was paramount. However, simultaneously, an acknowledgement that families were not always able to care for their own led to the development of social welfare structures to support children and the infirm when their families could not. These services were most often provided through religious institutions, although they were sometimes provided by local government.

Preoccupation with Childhood (Nineteenth Century to the Present)

As industrialization led to rapid changes in family structures, population growth, and urbanization, society shifted into a period of preoccupation with childhood that continues today. For much of history, it was incumbent on the family or religious groups to serve the needs of their own, including children. However, demographic changes and shifts in theoretical perspectives coincided to produce a new time period where children are seen as invaluable members of society. As people began to see children as persons with their own value and needs, society developed structures through which the specific needs of children would be met.

While the state and federal levels of government were not involved in the design or provision of social welfare policies or practices to support children and families until the middle of the nineteenth century, non-governmental, largely religiously affiliated institutions started to develop such services. These "voluntary" services began to spontaneously appear in different parts of the United States, usually led by convents, churches, or individual philanthropists who felt a moral, if not religious, obligation to assist the needy.

One such institution that saw a great expansion in use during this time period was the orphanage. Orphanages are largely believed to house children whose parents are deceased. However, many, if not most, orphans had at least one living parent. Since there was generally no outdoor relief available for poor families in the United States in the eighteenth and nineteenth centuries, a parent could place a child into an orphanage for temporary care, while s/he attempted to right her/his troubled financial circumstances. Many orphanages allowed or even encouraged parental contact with institutionalized children. Contrary to the conditions presented through popular culture (like the musical *Annie*), orphanages were not designed to place children without parents into new families. Instead, orphanages were structured environments where children were physically cared for until they reached an age at which they could be employed and meet their own needs.

The first orphanage in the United States, Ursaline Convent, was founded in 1727 in New Orleans, Louisiana. By 1800 there were only five orphanages in the country. These early orphanages were not so much the response to the beginning of a social movement, but localized responses to specific events, like disease or the Indian Wars. However, larger societal influences began to take hold. Therefore, by 1851 there were 77 orphanages. By 1900 there were 400 orphanages throughout the United States serving more than 100,000 children. The rapid growth in the number of orphanages in the latter half of the nineteenth century coincides with rapid industrialization, urbanization, and immigration in the United States.

The decline of the indenture system and a growing belief that institutionalization could solve social problems led to growth in the number of orphanages, asylums for the mentally ill, and other similar institutions. It was believed that congregate settings provided opportunities to control and correct social problems in individuals.

Orphanages were viewed as services to the community. As a result, African-American children were largely excluded from receiving the benefits orphanages provided for families. Instead, communities placed African-American children deemed in need of supervision in jails or reform schools, even though the children were not delinquents. Orphanages specifically designed to serve African-American children were developed in some areas of the country, but not all.

Dorothea Dix (1802–1887), a well-known historical figure of the time, was the leader of a movement to remove the mentally ill from poorhouses and rehouse them in specialized institutions. Dix's advocacy on behalf of the mentally ill revolutionized society's response to social welfare needs. She was instrumental in efforts to convince state and federal governments to fund asylums for the mentally ill. Her successes and failures were used as teachings for the child welfare movement that later sought funding from the same sources.

The Orphan Train Movement

By the middle of the nineteenth century, urban populations were growing due to the retreat of many Americans from rural, farming culture, the promise of jobs in urban factories, as well as the start of rapid immigration from Europe. One by-product of urbanization was an increased number of "street children". There was no right to public education until the early twentieth century. As a result, many children worked in factories and other industries. Many others roamed city streets in search of food, work, or trouble.

In 1853, Charles Loring Brace (1826–1890) founded the Children's Aid Society in New York City to respond to what he saw as the plight of these street children (Children's Aid, 2010). The Children's Aid Society provided housing and created industrial schools to teach young boys and girls useful trade skills. The Children's Aid Society became a notable spearhead for a mass system of forced emigration. Poor children from urban areas on the East Coast of the United States were transported via railroad trains to rural, farming areas in the Midwest. The process, which was referred to as "placing out", became known as the "Orphan Train" movement.

The process of placing out involved gathering 40–100 children at a time from orphanages and other urban service providers and sending them by the railroad to towns in the Midwest. Children were accompanied on these trips by "agents", who were adults who served as nurses and surrogate parents during the trip and provided order. While there was a process of approving a home for placement before the children's arrival, after placement there was little oversight to guarantee that children were cared for appropriately.

Advertisements disseminated in Midwest towns along the train route announced the impending arrival of "Homeless Children". Families were encouraged to come to local theaters, churches, and opera houses to see the children and help find them "good homes". It was expected that the children would be treated "in every way as members of the family". The children were supposed to be sent to school and church, and they were to be provided with appropriate clothing until they turned 18.

When children arrived in a given town, they were lined up on a stage or platform for inspection by interested families. Children were then selected on sight for placement. Some children were chosen due to their perceived physical ability to work on a family farm or work in a family house doing cooking and cleaning. Younger children might have been chosen by infertile couples seeking to start or grow their families. Children who were not selected were reloaded onto the train, and the process was repeated in the next town.

Supporters of the Orphan Train movement highlight the effort's successes. It removed children from chaotic or neglectful homes in overcrowded urban areas. There are many stories of grateful children who were placed through the process into families where they lived fruitful and fulfilling lives.

Critics of the movement point to the fact that many of the "orphans" were not orphans. Children were actually separated, perhaps through coercion, from living parents, siblings, and extended families. There are many stories of children who were abused or exploited through the placing-out process. Some children ran away from their placements.

Discrimination was also a common criticism of the Orphan Train movement. Systemic racism was evident. There were only a handful of orphanages that took in Black children. When they did, they were most likely segregated, such as the Colored Orphan Asylum in New York City. Though Black children and families were just as likely, if not more likely, to need social services in this time period, they were not included in the groups of children transported to the Midwest. There was speculation that White rural farming families of the Midwest would be less likely to open their homes to Black children. Additionally, the Orphan Train movement depended on the generosity of wealthy donors to cover program costs. It was believed that wealthy donors were less likely to contribute funds to efforts aimed at alleviating social problems for Black children. Thus, Black children were systematically denied any perceived benefits of the Orphan Train movement

In addition to racial discrimination, religious discrimination is consistently asserted as a basis for the design of the Orphan Train movement, and Catholic children were the movement's primary targets. In the mid-to-late nineteenth century, the largest groups of immigrants to urban areas on the East Coast were Roman Catholics from Germany, Ireland, and Italy. A significant movement led by Protestant Americans, the "Nativist" movement, argued that Catholics would ruin the existing culture of the United States. Charles Loring Brace has been credited with the belief that Catholic families were, by definition, improper environments for raising children (O'Connor, 2001). As Catholic communities in major urban areas in the United States grew and organized, they developed their own social service agencies designed to serve Catholic children within the community. Some of these Catholic agencies developed programs similar to those of the Children's Aid Society. They also placed out Catholic children, but only with Catholic families, in other parts of the country.

Orphan Train programs ceased in the late 1920s and early 1930s after local and state governments became more involved in efforts to ensure the welfare of children, and children were alternatively placed locally with foster families. It is estimated that over 250,000 children were ultimately relocated through the emigration movement.[1]

Mary Ellen Wilson, and the New York Society for the Prevention of Cruelty to Children (NYSPCC)

Prior to 1873, parents could expect little or no interference with how they treated their children, and they had few places to ask for help. The government left families alone to determine how to raise their own children. Abandoned children or true orphans became wards of churches or early social service providers. Families also chose to place their children into care, either temporarily or permanently. In an early form of foster care, orphans or impoverished children were placed in orphanages or with other families. However, the government was rarely involved in these processes.

As a result of the primacy of the family in determining how children were raised, there were no laws in place in the United States or any other country specifically outlining the rights and responsibilities of parents or children. Criminal prosecution was available in cases of egregious parental acts against children, but it was rarely used. The long-held societal belief that no one should interfere into the functioning of families began to rapidly erode in 1873, when the abuse of Mary Ellen Wilson (1864–1956) led to the creation of the first child welfare agency in the world, the New York Society for the Prevention of Cruelty to Children (NYSPCC).

Etta Wheeler (1834–1921) was a "friendly visitor" (early social worker) from St. Luke's Methodist Mission in New York City. As a friendly visitor, she walked around the neighborhood and met with members of her church's parish who needed food, assistance, or just company. During one such visit, a neighbor told her about a child she was concerned about. The neighbor had observed the barely dressed child locked out of the home in the cold. The neighbor also overheard the child's screams and believed the child was being beaten. With no formal mechanism to intervene with the family available at her own agency, or any other agency, Ms. Wheeler conducted a discreet investigation.

The child, Mary Ellen, was not in the custody of her biological parents. Her parents had never married. She was being cared for by her biological father's ex-wife, who had remarried. When Ms. Wheeler met with the family, she observed Mary Ellen as follows:

> I saw a pale, thin child, barefoot, in a thin, scanty dress so tattered that I could see she wore but one garment besides. It was December and the weather bitterly cold … Across the table lay a brutal whip of twisted leather strands and the child's meager arms and legs bore many marks of its use.
>
> (New York Society for the Prevention of Cruelty to Children, 2000)

Distraught by what she observed, Ms. Wheeler sought advice from anyone she could find. Eventually, she consulted a man well-known at the time for his strong position against the cruel treatment of work horses on the streets of New York City, Henry Bergh (1813–1888). Mr. Bergh had worked tirelessly to get passed in 1866 in New York State the first legislation in the country against animal cruelty.

In response to Ms. Wheeler's request for assistance, Mr. Bergh enlisted the help of a good friend and local attorney, Elbridge Gerry (1837–1927). Mr. Gerry creatively used an obscure section of the law to have Mary Ellen removed from the home and to prosecute Mary Ellen's caretaker. The case of Mary Ellen Wilson gained notoriety across the country and around the world. The trial of her caretaker was reported in newspapers from coast to coast and beyond. One prominent courtroom observer was Jacob Riis (1849–1914), a social reformer, photographer, and journalist. He wrote about the experience:

> I was in a courtroom full of men with pale, stern looks. I saw a child brought in ... at the sight of which men wept aloud. And as I looked, I knew I was where the first chapter of children's rights was written ... For from that dingy courtroom ... came forth The New York Society for the Prevention of Cruelty to Children with all it has meant to the world's life.
> (New York Society for the Prevention of Cruelty to Children, 2000)

In 1875, Bergh, Gerry, and others formed the New York Society for the Prevention of Cruelty Children (NYSPCC), the first child welfare organization in the world. The NYSPCC then developed the new role of investigating and prosecuting child abuse cases in New York City. Other Societies for the Prevention of Cruelty to Children (SPCCs) were formed across the country and around the world. SPCCs were private entities funded through donations from the wealthy.

Much like the animal protection agencies that Mr. Bergh also designed, SPCCs were empowered through the laws of individual states to receive reports of concerns, investigate cases, and refer complaints of child abuse to the relevant criminal court of the jurisdiction for prosecution. New York State was the first state to pass such a law. The laws empowered SPCCs to act on behalf of the State Attorney General or local District Attorney in abuse cases. In its first year of existence, the NYSPCC received several hundred reports of concerns, prosecuted almost 70 cases, and removed more than 70 children from abusive conditions in New York City alone.

Many SPCCs are still in existence today, including the NYSPCC. However, the role of the SPCCs has changed dramatically since their introduction over 130 years ago. As the role of government child protective services expanded in the mid-to-late twentieth century, SPCCs either adapted to provide other services to families and children or they became defunct.

Development of Private Social Child Welfare Organizations

The nineteenth century saw a large societal response to growing recognition of social problems, including mental illness, public health, and child maltreatment. The mechanisms developed to respond to issues came in the form of private agencies, not government intervention. Privately owned and incorporated social service agencies were created in the 1800s across the country. These agencies were most often funded through small groups of wealthy benefactors or well-supported religious organizations. Agencies were designed to address issues on the scale most appropriate to the funders' interests. As a result, small segments of larger communities or entire geographic areas were deprived of the resources afforded by private agencies. This phenomenon was experienced by the burgeoning child welfare movement.

In 1920 the United States Census found urban dwellers outnumbering rural dwellers. As could be expected, most of the private provision of social services was aimed at urban areas. By 1922, there were 300 SPCCs across the United States, largely in urban areas. Three hundred might seem like a large number, but there were over 100 million people living in the United States at that time.

Resulting Racial, Religious, and Ethnic Discrimination

Before the equal protection clause of the Constitution of the United States was applied to services provided by large private social service agencies by extension of the interstate commerce clause, nineteenth-century private agencies had the right to exclude anyone from receiving the services they provided. At the time, agencies were able to refuse service to individuals based on gender, race, religion, or immigration status, among other classifications. Groups that were determined less worthy, most often children of color, including African-American and Native American children, were systematically excluded from services specifically designed to address the problems poor children faced.

As previously discussed, African-American children were often excluded from orphanages. Additionally, they were rarely served by mental asylums. While SPCCs did not necessarily specifically articulate a refusal to serve African-American children, children of color identified for intervention were less likely to be placed in family foster care and more likely to be placed in reform schools and jails.

A report by Frances Blascoer (1915) entitled *Colored School Children in New York*, which was based on interviews with the heads of many private and government agencies, speaks of these phenomena. Ms. Blascoer was a former Settlement House Worker and the first Executive Secretary of the National Association for the Advancement of Colored People (NAACP). As a Special Investigator for the Committee on Hygiene of the Public Education Association of New York City, Blascoer wrote:

The Superintendent of the Society for the Prevention of Cruelty to Children said he had not much hope of rehabilitating colored girls of the type his society took into custody. He said they had no conception of morals and were so untruthful that he found it difficult to secure adequate testimony on which to convict men accused of harming them, even when he had corroborating testimony. He thought more work should be done to raise the morals of the race. There was apparently little trouble in placing delinquent colored boys, as the House of Refuge on Randall's Island could always be depended upon in any ordinary circumstances.

(Blascoer, 1915, p. 32)

Native American children received specialized attention in the provision of private and subsequent government-sponsored social services as well. Religious organizations, starting as early as the seventeenth century, established specialized schools for Native American children in an effort to convert them to Christianity. By the middle of the nineteenth century, the success of such schools led to significant growth in what came to be referred to as "Indian Boarding Schools". They were found throughout the rural countryside of the growing country.

Often Native American children were either enticed into matriculating into these institutions with false promises or required to enroll through the threat of physical force against whole communities. When children arrived at these schools, they were literally and figuratively stripped of their cultural identities. Long hair was cut. Children were assigned new "American" names. The expressed purpose of such methods was to start the process of assimilating children into "American" cultural and societal norms.

In 1877 there were 47 such schools in operation in the United States, serving more than 5,000 students. By 1900 there were nearly 150, mostly in the states of the Great Plains with substantial Native American communities. In the early twentieth century, state and federal governments ultimately took responsibility for financing and/or running these facilities under the Bureau of Indian Affairs. By the late 1920s, Indian Boarding Schools had fallen out of favor due to their high financial costs and changes in public education policies, which expanded free public education to include Native American children.

Religion was also a basis on which children were discriminated against, especially in the early child welfare system. As previously discussed, Catholic children were seen as a target for early child welfare interventions, including the Orphan Train movement. Jewish children, largely from immigrant families arriving from Eastern Europe, were also discriminated against, though not in the same high numbers as Catholic children. As in Catholic communities, once Jewish communities became organized and started pooling resources, specialized services were made available to Jewish children and families in need. In 1845 United Hebrew Charities was established in New York City as an umbrella organization for a handful of local Jewish community social service providers. Through a series of mergers and name changes, the organization morphed into its current form, the Jewish Board of Family and Children's Services. It is now the largest social services provider in New York State, serving all children regardless of religion or race.

Private, largely religiously affiliated social service agencies aimed at preserving child welfare have been primarily responsible for the development of social services in the United States. The structures they developed were replete with problems, including major gaps in service to specific communities and geographic areas. The eventual takeover of child welfare services by state and federal governments in the twentieth century aimed to universalize the provision of services regardless of race, religion, or ethnicity. However, the powerful stature of the individuals and organizations who created the original child welfare system influenced the resulting system, and the problematic provision of services continued in some jurisdictions, even up to today.

Early Government Involvement in Child Welfare

While private agencies were the largest providers of social services until the middle of the twentieth century, especially in the area of child welfare, there were many avenues through which local, state, and federal governments interceded or influenced policies and practices.

Child Labor

For many social reformers, their first entry into the area of child welfare was through efforts to reduce or eliminate child labor. In the early time periods discussed in this chapter, child labor was a given. Children's usefulness in society was largely determined by their ability to work on farms or in industry. As rapid industrialization gave way to factory jobs, working children provided families with an extra source of income and employers with a cheaper form of labor. As the United States entered the period of preoccupation with childhood, the first efforts to limit child labor can be seen in local- and state-level restrictions on the employment of children. Concerns about child welfare in dangerous factories coupled with concerns about low-cost child workers competing with adult workers resulted in a growing social movement to outlaw child labor.

By the middle of the nineteenth century, many states passed laws forbidding the employment of children under the age of 15, although the laws were rarely enforced. By the early twentieth century, the proliferation of labor unions, the progressive social reform movement, and their respective influence on policy resulted in large-scale child labor laws at the local and state levels as well as more consistent enforcement. While a constitutional amendment outlawing child labor was passed by Congress in 1920, it was not ratified and never went into effect.

Parallel to the movement to eliminate child labor was a movement to expand public education and require all children to complete a certain level of education. This movement, like the movement to eliminate child labor, had multiple motives. One early motive for compulsory education was religious organizations' desire to prepare children to be literate bible readers. Labor reformers saw compulsory education as a way to systematically remove children from the labor pool, leaving more jobs for adults. Some social reformers sought to use compulsory education to assimilate immigrant or Native American children. A later, larger motive founded in the progressive movement was to improve overall child outcomes.

By 1900, 34 states had compulsory education laws. By 1910, 72% of American children attended school. By 1918, every state required children to attain at least an elementary school education.

Juvenile Courts

The juvenile court system is a structure through which the government developed policies and practices aimed at ensuring the welfare of children. The country's first juvenile court, which was located in Cook County (Chicago), Illinois, was established through the Illinois Juvenile Court Act of 1899. Juvenile courts exercised the state's *parens patriae* (Latin for "parent of the nation") authority. This authority allows the government to step in for the judgment of parents as necessary to secure the well-being of children. It is a power used in child welfare proceedings as well.

It should come as no surprise that the Juvenile Court Act and juvenile courts largely resulted from the advocacy efforts of early social work pioneers, such as Jane Addams (1860–1935) and the supporters of her Hull House. Reformers sought to remove children who were responsible for criminal acts from the existing system's reform houses and jails. The aim was to separate child offenders from adult offenders, provide specialized services to rehabilitate children, and support their families in order to prevent future bad behavior. By 1925, juvenile courts had been established in all but two states.

The juvenile court system developed alongside the child welfare system. Juvenile courts provided children with specialized treatment that differed from what was afforded to adults. A series of court cases in the 1960s and 1970s highlighted how the separate and specialized system actually developed mechanisms to deny children rights that should have been afforded to them.

White House Conference on Children

In 1910, largely in response to growing recognition of the special needs of children and their families, the first White House Conference on Children took place in Washington, DC. It focused on the needs of dependent children in out-of-home care. The conference was called by President

Theodore Roosevelt after significant lobbying by Lillian Wald (1867–1940), a public health nurse and founder of the Henry Street Settlement in New York City, and Florence Kelley (1859–1932), another social reformer involved in the establishment of the NAACP. The meeting brought together social workers, educators, juvenile court judges, labor leaders, and civic-minded men and women concerned with the care of dependent children. Participants discussed policy initiatives and designed nine specific policy proposals that emphasized the importance of family, called for regular government inspections of foster-care homes, and supported education and medical care for children in foster care.

One of the major outcomes of the conference was the establishment of the United States Children's Bureau in 1912. Over the past century the Children's Bureau developed into the premier federal agency responsible for the care and welfare of children and families. It was responsible for policy initiatives aimed at addressing infant and maternal death, child labor, delinquency, family economic security, child maltreatment, and foster care.

After the initial conference, a White House Conference on Children was held every ten years for the next 60 years. Each focused on specific issues relevant to children in the time period. The last, hosted by President Nixon, took place in 1970.

Integration of Professional Social Work in the Development of Non-governmental Child Welfare Services

Not coincidentally, growth in the movement to secure child welfare parallels the introduction and expansion of the social work profession and related human services. In fact, training programs created to prepare workers for the Charitable Organization Society (COS) and settlement houses, networked across the country, were the basis for early social work education. Early training programs eventually moved from agencies to academia. Social work was taught in colleges and universities. From Jane Addams's Hull House to Mary Richmond (1861–1928) and her integral work with the COS, social work practice was integral to shaping society's response to the plight of impoverished families and children.

While New York City can claim the distinction of being the birthplace of the child welfare agency, through the NYSPCC, Boston is the city where child welfare practice was professionalized. The New York form of child welfare was largely modeled on law-enforcement policies and practices of the time. While some social work training programs were developed in New York City, they were aimed at preparing workers for jobs in local settlement houses, not in the SPCCs.

However, in the late nineteenth century, Boston child welfare reformers began applying Mary Richmond's methods of scientific charity to child protection. Parallel efforts by the Boston Children's Aid Society and the Massachusetts Society for the Prevention of Cruelty to Children resulted in methods designed to not just investigate, but also assess and evaluate children and families. These new methods sought to find and correct the reasons why families presented to agencies for intervention, instead of simply removing children and punishing caretakers.

Discovery of "Battered Child Syndrome"

For 50 years after the case of Mary Ellen Wilson, there was rapid and widespread growth in concern for and societal responses to children in need. The economic prosperity of the 1920s provided fewer incentives for investment in child welfare services. The economic depression of the 1930s and early 1940s and the country's subsequent involvement in World War II detracted attention from the plight of children. Instead, attention was focused on larger economic and national security interests.

In the middle of the twentieth century, however, there was a return to focusing on the needs of children, which resulted in a revolution in policies and practices that produced the child welfare system we know in the United States today. In the 1950s, groups of doctors began studying broken bones in children. With the increasing use of x-ray technology, doctors were better able to identify broken bones. In many cases, doctors saw older injuries as well as recent breaks when they looked at x-rays. Past injuries were often unexplained by the child and parents. Shocked by the possibility that parents could be harming their children in such a way, doctors conducted further research. In 1962, Dr. C. Henry Kempe and his colleagues published a seminal report in the *Journal of the American Medical Association* that introduced "Battered Child Syndrome", which was defined as "a clinical condition in young children who have received serious physical abuse, generally from a parent or foster parent" (Kempe et al., 1962, p. 17).

The response from society at large and policymakers, in particular, was impressive. That same year, the US Children's Bureau held a conference to draft model child welfare legislation, and the Social Security Act was amended to require states to make a plan to provide child protective services. In 1963, 11 of the 18 bills dealing with child abuse that were introduced in Congress were passed. By 1967, all 50 states had laws requiring certain professionals to report suspicions of child abuse.

Due to increasing recognition of child abuse as a serious problem in the United States in the twentieth century, the government took on investigative and prosecutorial roles in abuse cases, replacing the traditionally private provision of services through SPCCs. From the 1960s, individual state governments developed systems for responding to child abuse, often guided by suggestions from the federal government. The resulting state and federal system of child protection is the framework through which the current child welfare system is run. Chapter 3 explores policies related to government-run child welfare systems between the early 1960s through to the present day.

Case Examples and Questions

1   At the end of the US Civil War in 1865, there were nearly four million newly freed slaves. Reports suggest that almost half of these new citizens were children. A significant proportion of the freed children had been separated from their families or orphaned. Many remained in the South, mostly in rural areas. Freed Black children without caretakers were often relegated either to institutions or to the workforce. While freed Black children faced conditions similar to those experienced by immigrant Catholic children in urban areas on the East Coast, there were no Orphan Train-like "movements" to relocate emancipated children to better conditions. Why do you think there was a difference in the treatment of and provision of services to freed Black children compared to the children "served" by the Orphan Trains?

2   Research consistently finds that boys and girls have an equal likelihood of being abused and/or neglected.

   (A)   Do you think the societal response would have been the same if Etta Wheeler saved a boy instead of Mary Ellen Wilson?

   (B)   If you think the response would have been different, how? Why?

   (C)   What do you think the societal response would have been if Mary Ellen Wilson had been Black?

Note

1   A similar child transportation movement took place in Great Britain. In the early-to-mid twentieth century, children from church-sponsored orphanages were sent to live with families and in institutions in Australia. For a poignant and moving account of the "discovery" of this government-funded child deportation years after it ended and for touching stories of the families affected, read *Oranges and Sunshine* (originally titled *Empty Cradles*) by Margaret Humphreys or watch the 2010 motion picture by the same name.

Further Reading

For a great fictional account of the experience of children involved in the Orphan Train Movement, read *Orphan Train* by Christina Baker Kline, 2013.

Additional Resources

Marquis, C. (1996). The Rearing of Slave Children and Their Parental Relationships Before and After Emancipation. *Sloping Halls Review*, 3.

References

Blascoer, F. (1915). *Colored School Children in New York*. New York: Public Education Association of the City of New York, January 30.

Children's Aid. (2010). History. *Children's Aid*. Retrieved from: http://www.chil drensaidsociety.org/about/history.

Empey, L.T., Stafford, M.C., & Hay, C.H. (1999). *American Delinquency*, 4th edition. Belmont, CA: Wadsworth.

Humphreys, M. (1994). *Empty Cradles*. Sydney: Penguin Books.

Kempe, C.H., Silverman, F.N., Steele, B.F., Droegemueller, W., & Silver, H.K. (1962). The Battered-Child Syndrome. *Journal of the American Medical Association*, 181 (1), 17.

Kline, Christina Baker. (2013). *Orphan Train*. New York: Harper Collins.

New York Society for the Prevention of Cruelty to Children. (2000). *125th Anniversary Celebration Booklet*. New York: NYSPCC.

O'Connor, S. (2001). When Children Relied on Faith-Based Agencies. *New York Times*, May 26.

3 Child Welfare Policy
1960 to Present

Getting the Government Involved

Most social workers today presume that the government has a primary role in the provision of child welfare and child protection policy and services. When we think of Child Protective Services (CPS), we automatically think about state- or local-level governments responding to concerns related to child maltreatment. However, the CPS system that has existed throughout our lifetimes is actually relatively new in the larger scheme of government responsibility. Government-run CPS developed out of the growing societal recognition of child abuse in the 1960s.

The recognition of "Battered Child Syndrome" by medical professionals in the early 1960s resulted in a proliferation of high-impact media coverage that went beyond local newspapers. For instance, while local media outlets were known to cover stories about children who died at the hands of abusive parents, the national media rarely, if ever, covered these tragedies. After the identification of "Battered Child Syndrome", national news outlets (largely magazines such as *Newsweek, Time, Good Housekeeping*, and *Life*) ran stories that brought local news to the national spotlight (Myers, 2008).

In addition to impacting mainstream media reporting, the recognition of "Battered Child Syndrome" influenced academic research and writing as well (Kempe et al., 1962). Prior to 1962, there was little or no academic literature or research on child maltreatment. After the Kempe article, child maltreatment research and writing proliferated. A brief perusal of a 2014 list of peer-reviewed journals associated with social work reveals more than 15 items devoted to topics related to child maltreatment (Leung & Cheung, 2014).

With the medical and academic communities in sync with mainstream society's increasing concern with protecting children from harm at the hands of caretakers, there was pressure to change the societal response to child abuse and neglect. Amendments to the Social Security Act in 1962 included new language related to "Child Protective Services", which had not been part of the original 1935 Act. Specifically, the amendments called upon states to "pledge" to make child welfare services available statewide by

1975. Additionally, the amendments provided federal money to support the expansion of child welfare services (Myers, 2008).

As a result, states began usurping the role that had been held by SPCCs for nearly a hundred years. States take over responsibility for investigating allegations of child maltreatment, removing children from abusive homes, and placing children into orphanages or foster families. As a result, the first laws to actually address child abuse and neglect, which included the development of systems for mandated reporting (see Chapter 11), were designed at the state level (Lau et al., 2009). The federal government was barely involved. During a hearing in 1973, Walter Mondale, former United States Senator and 1984 Democratic presidential candidate, said: "[n]owhere in the Federal Government [can] we find one official assigned full time to the prevention, identification, and treatment of child abuse and neglect" (Mondale, 1974).

With 50 different states authoring independent legislation, there was a lot of variation in the language of laws across the country. Some states amended pre-existing statutes; some copied legislation passed by other jurisdictions; while others developed wholly new laws. Some states incorporated the new legislation in their penal or criminal laws, while others incorporated the legislation in general or welfare laws (Shephard, 1965).

In response, the federal government stepped in to encourage uniformity. Prompted by a decade's worth of research and feedback from professionals, the federal government passed the Child Abuse Prevention and Treatment Act of 1974 (1974), otherwise known as CAPTA.

Resulting Policies

Child Abuse Prevention and Treatment Act (CAPTA) of 1974

With CAPTA, the federal government influenced the role of CPS in individual states (Lau et al., 2009). The goal of CAPTA was to standardize child protection policies and practices across the states. Since states developed their own systems through the 1960s, definitions of child abuse and neglect varied widely from one state to another, as did the organization and structuring of CPS (Hutchison, 1993; Shephard, 1965). CAPTA provided the system that led to the relative uniformity in policy and practice that we experience with today's state and local CPS.

CAPTA led to uniformity largely through the efforts of the National Center for Child Abuse and Neglect (NCCAN) (Hutchison, 1993). NCCAN was established in order to develop model legislation for states to adopt. The model legislation defined child abuse, suggested organizational structures for agencies that receive reports of suspected abuse and neglect, and recommended a longer list of professionals who should be mandated to report suspected child abuse and neglect (Hutchison, 1993).

In the mid-1970s, NCCAN sponsored an advisory committee to develop the model legislation. The committee consisted primarily of lawyers, judges, doctors, academics, and representatives from policy think-tanks. Unfortunately, the advisory committee lacked participation from the public welfare workers who would ultimately run systems at the state level. Also missing from the advisory committee were professionals (other than doctors) who would be required to report suspected child abuse as a result of the legislation, such as social workers and educational personnel (Sussman & Cohen, 1975).

The work of the advisory committee led to the creation of NCCAN-sponsored model legislation that was ultimately adopted, with little adjustment, by all 50 states. The NCCAN model legislation broadened the definition of child abuse by including not only physical and emotional abuse, but also neglect and sexual abuse in the list of reportable cases (Hutchison, 1993). The NCCAN model legislation also expanded the role of mandated reporter by including law-enforcement, educational, social-service, and mental-health personnel on the list of mandated reporters.

Perhaps most importantly, the NCCAN advisory committee was also charged with identifying the state-level agency that should receive and investigate allegations of child maltreatment. Law enforcement, juvenile courts, and departments of social service were the three state-level agencies that the advisory committee considered making responsible for receiving and responding to reports of child maltreatment (Indiana's Statutory Protection for the Abused Child, 1974; Sussman & Cohen, 1975).

There were many reasons why the NCCAN advisory committee considered law enforcement an appropriate spearhead for child abuse reporting and investigation. For instance, many forms of child maltreatment were already under the purview of law enforcement, such as sexual abuse and severe physical abuse. The police were already staffed around the clock every day of the year, so infrastructures were already available. Additionally, American citizens were already accustomed to calling local police for help, so another system would not have to be learned. However, there were concerns that the police lacked the ability to provide therapeutic resources to afflicted families and fears that criminal penalties would deter reporting (Sussman & Cohen, 1975).

The juvenile courts at the time were deemed inappropriate because the investigative role was not seen as fitting for a court. Since the courts ultimately decide the validity of allegations, they should not also be responsible for their investigation. Additionally, the juvenile courts of the era were busy responding to numerous United States Supreme Court decisions, which were drastically changing their way of practice. The cases were making juvenile courts reflect the more rigid standards of practice found in criminal courts. For instance, the Court's 1967 decision in *In Re Gault* (387 U.S. 1) provided those accused of juvenile delinquency many rights previously denied to them, including the right to counsel and the right against self-incrimination. There were concerns about adding additional responsibilities to juvenile courts already undergoing change in the time period (Sussman & Cohen, 1975).

Instead, the NCCAN determined that a state's department of social services was the most appropriate venue for receiving and investigating reports of child maltreatment. It was assumed that these departments would be best able to develop specialized offices for child protective services. Departments were expected to provide social services or treatment to families in need of intervention. The department of social services was seen as a non-punitive option. The goal was for reporters and families to see the department of social services as offering help, not just punishing wrongdoing (Sussman & Cohen, 1975).

However, there were concerns that, since departments of social services were already viewed as the "poor people's agency", child maltreatment might, as a result, be perceived as a problem exclusively of the poor (Sussman & Cohen, 1975). It is a continuing concern (Jonson-Reid et al., 2009).

By the time model legislation had been proffered by the federal government in the 1970s, more than half of the states were already operating under a model where reports of suspected child abuse were received by the state's department of social services (Sussman & Cohen, 1975). Currently, in most states CPS continues to be housed in a social services department on the state level (Lau et al., 2009).

If you remember your social welfare policy classes, you should be scratching your head here. What about the separate roles of the federal and state governments? Due to the separations in the roles of state and federal governments outlined in the United States Constitution, the federal government cannot force states to adopt suggestions in certain areas of law. Child welfare and education are two areas where the federal government cannot impose its requirements on the states. In order to "encourage" states to follow federal preferences, incentive systems were designed.

States that conformed to the NCCAN model legislation were rewarded with federal money to support state child protection services (Hutchison, 1993). Largely as a result of the financial incentives, by 1980 most states passed all model legislation promulgated by the NCCAN. Adoption of NCCAN model legislation resulted in increased uniformity across states at the time. Subsequent changes in state laws over the 20 years following initial adoption have resulted again in some variability across states, though much less so than before the federal efforts.

Starting with the Child Abuse Prevention and Treatment Act (CAPTA) of 1974, the federal government continued influencing the role of child protective services in individual states. CAPTA was reauthorized regularly over the past 30 years, with the most recent reauthorization occurring in 2010 (Child Abuse and Treatment Act of 2010, 2010). At each reauthorization, amendments were made in an effort to improve the system and reflect the current concerns for the system.

The overall purpose of CAPTA, over the years, has been to provide federal funding and guidance to states to support efforts at prevention, assessment, investigation, prosecution, and treatment of all forms of child maltreatment. CAPTA also helps guide federal support for research, evaluation, and data collection activities. Additionally, it provides grants to public and non-profit agencies for demonstration programs and projects (Child Welfare Information Gateway, 2017).

Indian Child Welfare Act of 1978

Concerns were quickly raised, especially related to racial injustice, as federal attention was increasingly directed at child protection systems that had historically worked at the local and state levels. In the early 1970s, after nearly 200 years of systematic racism against American Indians, the federal government started to reconcile past policies and practices with laws aimed at preserving and enhancing tribal sovereignty. With greater awareness of the needs of children and families, the federal government began to recognize the continuing injustices specifically suffered by American Indian families (see Chapter 2). Congress began a process through which the Indian Child Welfare Act (ICWA) of 1978 (25 U.S.C. § 1902) was ultimately devised and passed into law.

During the hearings that led to the passage of the ICWA, disturbing testimony was shared. For instance, the Association of American Indian Affairs presented the results of a study that found that 35% of *all* American Indian children were in out-of-home care in 1977. Even more distressing, approximately 85% of the children were placed with non-American Indian families (Byler, 1977). Congress realized the gravity of the situation and quickly passed the ICWA.

The goal of the ICWA was to "protect the best interests of Indian children and to promote the stability and security of Indian tribes and families" (Indian Child Welfare Act of 1978, 1978). The ICWA set forth federal guidelines for state child custody proceedings involving American Indian children, even outside the confines of child abuse and neglect cases. The ICWA required caseworkers to make special considerations when qualifying American Indian children were involved in their cases. Under the law case workers are held to a higher standard of providing active efforts to the family. For instance, when out-of-home placement was determined to be necessary, placement had to meet special requirements, such as it had to reflect the values of the child's culture. The standard to terminate the rights of American Indian parents was set at beyond a reasonable doubt, a higher threshold than the standard applied to any other parents. Additionally, the ICWA outlines ways for the CPS to communicate with tribal governments, including a requirement that tribal governments be notified if a child from a tribal community was removed from a home in order to facilitate the identification of an appropriate placement within the community (Child Welfare Information Gateway, 2003).

ICWA has long been considered a "gold standard" in child welfare policy (Child Welfare League of America, 2015). Following some of the successes of ICWA, similar policies were implemented with other children and families, like efforts to encourage out-of-home placements with family members.

Unfortunately, even 40 years later American Indian children and families continue to be disproportionately involved in the child welfare system. American Indian children are more likely to be victims of substantiated maltreatment as compared to all other children except African-American children. American Indian children are nearly three times more likely than white children to be in foster care (Maher et al., 2015).

As recently as 2015, a federal court found that South Dakota officials were removing American Indian children without evidence of child maltreatment and disproportionately placing them with non-American Indian foster families. Hundreds of children were removed from their homes. Every single subsequent hearing to challenge the removals led to a reversal of the CPS decision, and the children returned home after devastatingly unnecessary stays in foster care. A federal court judge ordered the state of South Dakota to take corrective action. The state failed to do so. In response the judge followed with a formal injunction against the discriminatory actions, which ensured that a continued failure to comply would result in contempt of court violations (*Oglala Sioux Tribe and Rosebud Sioux Tribe v. Fleming et al.*, 2016).

It is clear that more work needs to be done to prevent child maltreatment amongst American Indian families while protecting these communities from discriminatory policies and practices. One federal law is not nearly sufficient.

Adoption Assistance and Child Welfare Act of 1980 (AACWA)

Everyone knows that a single piece of federal legislation is never the solution. That is why even longstanding federal laws, like the Social Security Act, are consistently updated through amendments. Shortly after the enactment of CAPTA some serious flaws were recognized.

While it was a great idea to provide federal funding to state-run CPS, it essentially created an incentive system for removing children from their families and keeping them in foster care. States received more money to support a child removed from a family and placed into substitute care compared to the funding provided for prevention services to keep a child safely at home or funding for finding a permanent placement through adoption. There were no subsidies for children who were adopted, so foster parents lost financial support if they adopted a child in their care. As a result, the number of children in foster care rapidly increased in the first few years after CAPTA. The number of foster children in 1979 was double the number in care in 1960 (Barden,1979).

In response, the federal government designed and passed the Adoption Assistance and Child Welfare Act (AACWA) of 1980. President Jimmy Carter signed the Act into law. The AACWA is technically another amendment to the Social Security Act, but the AACWA added some important pieces to child welfare law that social workers still work with today. The AACWA established the requirement that CPS make "reasonable efforts" to keep children with their families. If a child could not safely remain with family, then CPS must make "reasonable efforts" to return a child to the family. How would CPS do this? Through the new concept of "permanency planning" (Child Welfare Information Gateway, 2003).

The AACWA set forth a series of requirements for periodic case reviews. Reviews occurred at least every six months while a child was in out-of-home care. In addition, a court hearing was required when a child was in out-of-home care for 18 months or more. The AACWA also provided federally funded adoption subsidies in an effort to encourage and increase the adoption of children with special needs and older children. Like CAPTA, AACWA instituted provisions through a series of reimbursements for state-level expenditures (Vandervort, 2010).

Title IV-E of the Social Security Act within the AACWA was of critical importance to the social work profession. Title IV-E provided open-ended federal funding to states for certain administrative and training activities.

Initially the AACWA had a substantial impact. By 1982 the number of children in foster care, around 250,000, began to decline. Then things changed. Ronald Reagan replaced Jimmy Carter in the presidency. The Congress elected along with Reagan was considerably more fiscally conservative than the previous one. As a result, many of the economic supports provided by the federal government to the states were rolled back. However, the requirements for practice were not. There were growing demands on child welfare services as the result of social problems related to substance use and HIV/AIDS. Foster care populations started increasing again. By 1993 the number of children in foster care in the United States was 464,000 and growing (Vandervort, 2010).

Title IV-E

From the first federal spending on child welfare in the early 1960s through 1980, federal funding was distributed through the Aid to Families with Dependent Children (AFDC) welfare program. The AACWA changed the funding mechanism. Starting in 1980, much of the federal support for child welfare was disseminated through Title IV-E of the Social Security Act (Office of the Assistant Secretary for Planning and Evaluation, US DHHS, 2005).

Since the late 1980s, Title IV-E funding has been used by states to support the education of social workers to prepare them careers in child welfare. Title IV-E funding is available to train current or future child welfare staff. In 2010, 147 BSW and MSW programs in 35 different states were financially able to support students pursuing a social work education thanks to Title IV-E funding (Social Work Policy Institute, 2012).

Adoption and Safe Families Act of 1997 (ASFA)

When considering the context for the Adoption and Safe Families Act of 1997 (ASFA), it is important to recognize the larger political landscape of the early-to-mid 1990s. President Ronald Reagan's two terms saw reduced federal spending and dramatic decreases in personal and corporate tax rates. President George H.W. Bush promised more of the same when he infamously pledged, "Read My Lips: No New Taxes". But the fiscal realities of the changing economy found President Bush supporting a budget with tax increases. His shift in fiscal position combined with competition in the 1992 presidential election from a strong third-party presidential candidate, Ross Perot, allowed the moderate Democratic southern governor, Bill Clinton, to eke out an electoral college win to secure the presidency.

While running for president, Clinton pledged to "End Welfare as We Know It". He followed through on his pledge. After compromising with the first Republican majority in the House of Representatives in 40 years, the Personal Responsibility and Work Opportunity Reconciliation Act (PRWORA) of 1996 was passed. It secured President Clinton a second term. The PRWORA eliminated many of the entitlements the federal government had developed over the years to help support poor people. Namely, the PRWORA ended the guaranteed support of Aid to Families with Dependent Children (AFDC). Temporary Assistance for Needy Families (TANF), which was put in its place, imposed time limits and work requirements to reduce "welfare dependency" and, thus, reduce the federal government's fiscal responsibility to support the poor.

Your social welfare policy textbooks provide more in-depth information about the development and aftermath of the PRWORA. For the purposes of the present child welfare policy discussion, it is important to note that the same Congress passed the ASFA into law in 1997. Congress was as focused on transforming child protection and child welfare policy as it was interested in ending entitlements to welfare, and it used some of the same policy devices to accomplish its goals.

The ASFA was largely developed in response to the growing numbers of children in foster care. At a time when unfunded prevention and family preservation programs were coupled with the crack cocaine epidemic of the 1980s and 1990s, state child protective systems were inundated with reports of suspected child maltreatment. Children were staying in foster care for an average of three years, and only 10% were adopted out of the system

(Adoption and Safe Families Act of 1997, 1997). With nearly half a million children in foster care, there was bi-partisan pressure to make changes to the child welfare system. The ASFA was that change.

The stated goals of the ASFA were to reduce the length of time children stayed in foster care and establish performance standards for child welfare practice at the state level. The ASFA created a system that financially penalized states if they could not show they were meeting the new standards (Phillips & Mann, 2013).

One of the new standards put a time limit on placing a child in foster care, which was intended to encourage the child's return home to the parent(s) within a set period of time. If a child was in out-of-home placement for 18 out of the last 22 months, the state was required to file a termination of parental rights petition, unless it could cite exceptional circumstances, in order to free the child up for adoption. In other words, if a parent was not ready to have a child returned to their care within roughly two years of initial foster care placement, then the child would not be returned to them at all (Phillips & Mann, 2013). The ASFA time limit on reunification is very similar to the PRWORA time limit on the receipt of TANF benefits.

In order to create secure foster care placements that could lead to adoption, caseworkers were required to work simultaneously towards *two* different goals for all children in out-of-home placement (Phillips & Mann, 2013). For instance, if a child was placed in foster care due to parental substance abuse, the primary plan might be reunification, but the secondary plan might be adoption. The child welfare worker was required to meet performance standards while working towards *both* plans: reunification and adoption (New York State Child Welfare Court Improvement Project, n.d.).

The ASFA also required a yearly court or administrative review of every case in which a child was in out-of-home placement. Almost all states instituted more formally structured case-level administrative and court-involved review processes. For instance, New York State requires court hearings at least once every six months when a child is in out-of-home placement, while Virginia and Georgia require such hearings every four months (Child Welfare Information Gateway, 2016).

States were audited by the federal government at regular intervals. If states were unable to show that they were meeting the ASFA requirements, they suffered financial punishments. Reimbursement of funds for state child welfare systems were reduced if they were found to be substantially out of compliance (more than 10%) with the ASFA standards. For instance, New York State passed its primary foster care review in 2006 after fewer than 9% of the 110 cases randomly sampled for review were found to be out of compliance with the ASFA standards (New York State Child Welfare Court Improvement Project, n.d.).

There is no denying that the ASFA made an indelible impact on child protection and child welfare policies and practices across the United States.

While the ASFA alone should not be credited with the reduction in the number of children in foster care after 1997, there is no doubt that child welfare practice in the United States was revolutionized through its pressures for timely reunification, its call for securing alternative permanent plans for children, and its increased emphasis on proper case management. Unfortunately, one of the negative impacts of the ASFA was an increase in the termination of parental rights, specifically for incarcerated parents (Lee et al., 2005).

Family First Prevention Services Act of 2008 (FFPSA)

The Family First Prevention Services Act (FFPSA) ushered in some of the biggest changes to the structure of federal child welfare finance since the 1980s. The FFPSA's goal was to provide additional federal resources to help families in crisis stay together by funding resources and support while the family is still together. In response to growing concerns about the conditions in congregate care placements for children, such as group homes, the law limited federal funding for these services. The law also included several other child welfare-related updates to federal policy.

Future of Child Welfare Policy

Unfortunately, child welfare policy is not always a priority for any level of government at any given time. When the economy is in crisis or when other policy issues garner the attention of the larger population, the needs of children and families are too often ignored by policymakers.

As this text goes to print, the United States is at the center of the COVID-19 pandemic. Children across the country are learning from home. Millions of parents are out of work. The economic consequences of the COVID-19 crisis are clearly the priority for policymakers at all levels. The voice of social work is needed now more than ever.

It is imperative that social workers make the policy needs of children and families a priority. We share a knowledge of our history and tools for analysis and advocacy. Social workers could be responsible for the next important policy that will shape the future of the child welfare system.

Case Examples and Questions

1   While the policy discussion throughout the chapter rarely references race or ethnicity, it is important to recognize that children of color are disproportionately involved in the child welfare system.

   (A)   What role do you think federal policies played in racial disproportionality in the current child welfare system?

(B)   What role, if any, do you think race and ethnicity played in the development of the policies outlined in the chapter?

2   In the wake of the crack cocaine epidemic of the 1980s and 1990s, huge numbers of children entered and remained in foster care. More recently, the United States has experienced an epidemic of opioid addiction, which has similarly impacted the number of children in foster care.

(A)   How can policymakers learn from the experiences of the past to better respond to the current crisis?

(B)   The "face" of the crack epidemic was black, while the "face" of the opioid epidemic is white. What differences do you see in the ways various levels of government responded to the epidemics?

References

Adoption and Safe Families Act of 1997 (1997). H.R. 867, 105th Congress, November 19.

Barden, J.C. (1979). System of Foster Care for Children Assailed as Flawed and Costly: Total Doubled Since 1960. *New York Times*, April 24, A17.

Byler, W. (1977). *Statistical Survey of Out of Home Placement of Indian Children*. New York: Association on American Indian Affairs.

Child Abuse Prevention and Treatment Act of 1974 (1974). Public Law 93–247, January 31.

Child Abuse Prevention and Treatment Act of 2010 (2010). Public Law 111–320, December 12.

Child Welfare Information Gateway. (2003). *Major Federal Legislation Concerned with Child Protection, Child Welfare, and Adoption*. Washington, DC: US Department of Health and Human Services, Children's Bureau.

Child Welfare Information Gateway. (2016). *Court Hearings for the Permanent Placement of Children*. Washington, DC: US Department of Health and Human Services, Children's Bureau.

Child Welfare Information Gateway. (2017). *About CAPTA: A Legislative History*. Washington, DC: US Department of Health and Human Services, Children's Bureau.

Child Welfare League of America. (2015). *New Regulations to Improve the Indian Child Welfare Act Proceedings*. Washington, DC: Child Welfare League of America.

Hutchison, E.D. (1993). Mandatory Reporting Laws: Child Protective Case Finding Gone Awry? *Social Work*, 38 (1), 56–63.

Indian Child Welfare Act of 1978 (1978). 25 U.S.C. § 1902. Public Law 95–608, November 8.

Indiana's Statutory Protection for the Abused Child. (1974). *Valparaiso University Law Review*, 9 (1), 89–133. Retrieved from: https://scholar.valpo.edu/vulr/vol9/iss1/4.

In Re Gault, 387 U.S. 1 (1967).

Jonson-Reid, M., Drake, B., & Kolh, P.L. (2009). Is the Overrepresentation of the Poor in Child Welfare Caseloads Due to Bias or Need? *Children and Youth Services Review*, 31 (3): 422–427.

Kempe, C.H., Silverman, F.N., Steele, B.F., Droegemueller, W., & Silver, H.K. (1962). The Battered-Child Syndrome. *Journal of the American Medical Association*, 181 (1), 17.

Lau, K., Morse, R., & Krase, K. (2009). *Mandated Reporting of Child Abuse and Neglect: A Practical Guide for Social Workers*. New York: Springer Publishing Company.

Lee, A.F., Genty, P.M., & Laver, M. (2005). *The Impact of the Adoption and Safe Families Act on Children of Incarcerated Parents*. Washington, DC: Child Welfare League of America.

Leung, P.L. & Cheung, M. (2014). Journals in Social Work and Related Disciplines Manuscript Submission Information. *University of Houston*. Retrieved from: https://uh.edu/socialwork/_docs/cwep/journalsImpactFactorsHIndex.pdf.

Maher, E.J., Clyde, M., Darnell, A., Landsverk, J., & Zhang, J. (2015). Placement Patterns of American Indian Children Involved with Child Welfare. *Casey Family Programs*. Retrieved from: https://www.casey.org/media/NSCAW-Placement-Patterns-Brief.pdf.

Mondale, W. (1974). Letter of Transmittal to Harrison A. Williams, March 15. *Questions and Answers on Children and Youth of the Committee on Labor and Public Welfare, United States Senate*, 93rd Congress, 2nd Session, Part VII.

Myers, J.E.B. (2008). A Short History of Child Protection in America, *Family Law Quarterly*, 42 (3): 449–463.

New York State Child Welfare Court Improvement Project. (n.d.). *Best Practices Bulletin*. New York State Unified Court System: Division of Court Operations, Office of Alternative Dispute Resolution and Court Improvement Programs.

Office of the Assistant Secretary for Planning and Evaluation, US DHHS. (2005). Federal Foster Care Financing: How and Why the Current Funding Structure Fails to Meet the Needs of the Child Welfare Field. Background and History of Title IV-E Foster Care. *ASPE: Office of the Assistant Secretary for Planning and Evaluation*. Retrieved from: https://aspe.hhs.gov/report/federal-foster-care-financing-how-and-why-current-funding-structure-fails-meet-needs-child-welfare-field/background-and-history-title-iv-e-foster-care.

Oglala Sioux Tribe and Rosebud Sioux Tribe v. Fleming et al. (2016). United States District Court, District of South Dakota, Western Division, Civ. 13–5020-JLV

Phillips, C.M. & Mann, A. (2013). Historical Analysis of the Adoption and Safe Families Act of 1997. *Journal of Human Behavior in the Social Environment*, 23: 862–868.

Shephard, R.E. (1965). The Abused Child and the Law. *Washington & Lee Law Review*, 22 (2), 182–195.

Social Work Policy Institute. (2012). *Educating Social Workers for Child Welfare Practice: The Status of Using Title IV-E Funding to Support BSW and MSW Education*. Washington, DC: National Association of Social Workers.

Sussman, A. & Cohen, S. (1975). *Reporting Child Abuse and Neglect: Guidelines for Legislation*. Cambridge, MA: Ballinger Publishing Company.

Vandervort, F. (2010). Federal child welfare legislation. In D.N. Duquette & A.M. Haralambie (Eds.), *Child Welfare Law and Practice: Representing Children, Parents, and State Agencies in Abuse, Neglect, and Dependency Cases*, 2nd edition, 199–230. Denver, CO: Bradford Pub. Co.

4 Using Theory to Understand Child Maltreatment

Introduction to Theory in Child Welfare

Theory can be defined as an attempt to explain an occurrence. In the case of this textbook, we are focusing on theory as it relates to child abuse and neglect. Theory, in general, relates to objective facts that can be agreed upon by all observers. Even though theory relates to objective facts, theory itself is subjective. You can argue for or against theories, therefore they are not facts.

In this textbook, theories on the subject of child maltreatment relate to why child maltreatment occurs and why child maltreatment occurs in certain, but not all, families. Theory in general and theories on the subject of child abuse and neglect in particular rarely satisfy all readers or provide a complete explanation for an occurrence. Child abuse and neglect are not mathematics, physics, or chemistry. Child abuse and neglect happen to people. People are more complex than numbers, mass, or atoms. With this in mind, the theories offered in this chapter are to help social work students consider various perspectives on the causes of child maltreatment. Theory can inform assessment, intervention, and advocacy to prevent child maltreatment before it occurs, and theory can shape responses to and the treatment of victims and perpetrators of child maltreatment after it has been identified.

Social Learning Theory

Social learning theory suggests that people learn behavior by observing behavior in others, a phenomenon known as "modeling" (Bandura et al., 1961).

Social learning theory supports the concept of intergenerational "transmission" of child maltreatment. Intergenerational theory suggests that parents who mistreat their children were mistreated as children themselves. Risk factor analysis confirms that parents who mistreat their children are more likely to have been victims of child maltreatment. However, the limitations of social learning theory are readily apparent. Parents who maltreat their children were not all child victims themselves. Similarly, children who are maltreated do not all go on to mistreat their own children. Additional theories have attempted to fill the gap in social learning theory.

Attachment Theory

Research suggests that children with secure attachments are less likely to be abused or neglected by their caretakers (Capaldo & Perrella, 2018). According to attachment theory, connections between human beings developed through an evolutionary process in order to ensure survival (Bowlby, 1958). For instance, infants with firm attachments to their mothers were more likely to survive because their mothers were more likely to ensure the infants' protection.

Ainsworth and Bell (1970) developed a procedure for evaluating the attachment between child and parent, which was characterized by one of three categories: secure attachment, resistant attachment, or avoidant attachment. Children with a secure attachment to a parent/caretaker show confidence that their needs will be met through the relationship. Children with a resistant attachment to a parent/caretaker may seem to be independent, and when distressed they do not seek out assistance or comfort from the parent/caretaker. Children with an avoidant attachment may cling to the parent/caretaker, but they do not experience comfort as a result of the parental/caretaker interactions. When they are distressed, the parent/caretaker may be unable to soothe them.

Family Systems Theory

General systems theory was outlined by Ludwig von Bertalanffy (1968), who was attempting to explain how organisms interact with their environments. The work of von Bertalanffy was extrapolated into the fields of mathematics, sociology, and ultimately psychology/social work, where it was used to understand how groups, like families, function.

Family systems theory centers on the interrelatedness of family members. The actions of a family member cannot be understood in isolation. They must be examined within the context of the family as a system. The family, understood through the lens of family systems theory, is a system of interrelated parts. If one of the parts changes, the system will respond.

You may already be familiar with some of the key terms related to general and family systems theory: "boundaries", "homeostasis", "feedback loops", and "adaptation". "Boundaries" define the limits to a system. In the context of a family, boundaries can be defined by relationships. "Homeostasis" relates to the condition where the system maintains a certain level of function or balance. In the case of families experiencing child maltreatment, homeostasis may not be a healthy level of functioning. In that case, the goal of working with the family would be to support healthy "adaptation". "Adaptation" relates to a change in behavior, which forces the system to adjust and find a new form of homeostasis. Interventions by social workers or child protective services do not automatically result in healthy "adaptation". Instead, interventions should be seen as a form of a "feedback loop" that aims to support adaptation and new system conditions to result in a new, healthier state of "homeostasis".

Family systems theory focuses on the functioning of the family as a unit, instead of focusing on the problematic behavior of a particular member of the family. Family systems theory can explain why and how certain stressors on a family system may result in child maltreatment. Some stressors on a family system, like serious illness, unemployment, financial problems, or relationship problems, may be risk factors for child maltreatment.

Ecological Systems Theory

Ecological systems theory was designed by Urie Bronfenbrenner (1979) to explain how children are impacted by the systems that they interact with. The theory acknowledges various levels of influence over a child, including the microsystem, mesosystem, exosystem, macrosystem, and chronosystem levels.

The microsystem is the smallest level in the system and the closest to the child. The microsystem level includes the child's home environment, school/daycare, peer group, and other closely related contacts. The meso-system level involves connections between the microsystems in a child's environment. The exosystem level involves the connections between two systems where one system is found in the child's micro level of functioning and the other does not have a direct connection to the child. The macro-system level includes cultural patterns and community-level values as well as the political and economic systems that define other systems. The chronosystem level recognizes that the various systems involved in a child's life may vary or change over time, in part due to the individual's changing needs and development as well as because of changes in society.

Ecological systems theory presents a complex model for understanding how a child's development is impacted by various forces. The theory allows for additional theoretical context. For instance, interactional theory expands on ecological systems theory and focuses on interactions between children and parents as an influence on the likelihood of maltreatment (Belsky, 1980). The sociocultural context relates to concerns that acceptance of interpersonal violence at various system levels increases the likelihood of child maltreatment (Staub, 1996).

Ecological systems theory is explored further in Chapter 16.

Trauma-Informed Theory and Practice

The seminal Adverse Childhood Experiences (ACE) study highlighted the statistical connection between childhood trauma and negative outcomes in adulthood (Felitti et al., 1998). As a result, over the past 22 years trauma-informed theory and practice has aimed to mitigate the impact of child-hood adversity by supporting and enhancing resilience and recovery (Bunting et al., 2019).

Social workers who appreciate trauma-informed theory and utilize trauma-informed care neither ignore nor dwell on past trauma. Trauma-informed social workers are sensitive to how clients' current struggles are best understood in the context of their trauma experiences. Trauma-informed social workers start by validating the client's experiences, then they help trauma survivors understand how past experiences influence present circumstances.

Trauma-informed social work practiced with both victimized children and adults can mitigate the future risk of maltreatment to others as well as reduce the likelihood of negative outcomes for the victims themselves.

Case Examples and Questions

1   Consider the case of Mary Ellen Wilson discussed in Chapter 2, which resulted in the creation of the child welfare system. How can each of the following theories be used to better explain the conditions under which she was found? How can the theories be used to inform treatment of the child and family to mitigate long-term consequences from the abuse and neglect?

   (A)   Social learning theory
   (B)   Attachment theory
   (C)   Family systems theory
   (D)   Ecological systems theory
   (E)   Trauma-informed theory and practice

2   Consider the crisis of immigrant children and families detained in confinement camps on the border between the United States and Mexico. Many of these children have been separated from parents and siblings. How can each of the following theories be used to explain the harm that children experience as a result of their treatment in the confinement camps? And, how can the theories be used to inform treatment of the child and family to mitigate long-term consequences they may suffer as a result of their confinement?

   (A)   Social learning theory
   (B)   Attachment theory
   (C)   Family systems theory
   (D)   Ecological systems theory
   (E)   Trauma-informed theory and practice

References

Ainsworth, M.D.S. & Bell, S.M. (1970). Attachment, Exploration, and Separation: Illustrated by the Behavior of One-Year-Olds in a Strange Situation. *Child Development*, 41, 49–67.

Bandura, A., Ross, D., & Ross, S.A. (1961). Transmission of Aggression through Imitation of Aggressive Models. *The Journal of Abnormal and Social Psychology*, 63 (3), 575–582.

Belsky, J. (1980). Child Maltreatment: An Ecological Integration. *American Psychologist*, 35 (4), 320–335.

Bowlby, J. (1958). The Nature of the Child's Tie to His Mother. *International Journal of Psycho-analysis*, 39, 350–373.

Bronfenbrenner, U. (1979). *The Ecology of Human Development*. Cambridge, MA: Harvard University Press.

Bunting, L., Montgomery, L., Mooney, S., MacDonald, M., Coulter, S., Hayes, D., & Davidson, G. (2019). Trauma Informed Child Welfare Systems—A Rapid Evidence Review. *International Journal of Environmental Research and Public Health*, 16 (13), 2365.

Capaldo, M. & Perrella, R. (2018). Child Maltreatment: An Attachment Theory Perspective. *Mediterranean Journal of Clinical Psychology*, 6 (1).

Felitti, V.J., Anda, R.F., Nordenberg, D., Williamson, D.F., Spitz, A.M., Edwards, V., & Marks, J.S. (1998). Relationship of Childhood Abuse and Household Dysfunction to Many of the Leading Causes of Death in Adults: The Adverse Childhood Experiences (ACE) Study. *American Journal of Preventive Medicine*, 14 (4), 245–258.

Staub, E. (1996). Cultural-Societal Roots of Violence: The Examples of Genocidal Violence and of Contemporary Youth Violence in the United States. *American Psychologist*, 51 (2), 117–132.

von Bertalanffy, L. (1968). General Systems Theory as Integrating Factor in Contemporary Science. *Akten des XIV: Internationalen Kongresses für Philosophie*, 2, 335–340.

Part II
Defining Child Maltreatment

Child maltreatment is a global issue. However, many countries do not have laws about child maltreatment, and not all countries collect data about child maltreatment (World Health Organization, 2016). Because there are no universal definitions of child maltreatment used worldwide, estimates of the global scope of the problem vary widely (World Health Organization, 2016).

The World Health Organization (WHO) defines child maltreatment as "abuse and neglect that occurs to children under 18 years of age" (World Health Organization, 2016). The WHO definition includes

> all types of physical and/or emotional ill-treatment, sexual abuse, neglect, negligence and commercial or other exploitation, which results in actual or potential harm to the child's health, survival, development, or dignity in the context of a relationship of responsibility, trust, or power.
>
> (World Health Organization, 2016)

The WHO definition also sometimes includes "exposure to intimate partner violence" (World Health Organization, 2016, para. 2).

In the United States, child maltreatment is defined and reported through individual categories of conduct, including child abuse and neglect. The federal Child Abuse Prevention and Treatment Act (CAPTA) defines child abuse and neglect as "any recent act or failure to act on the part of a parent or caretaker which results in death, serious physical or emotional harm, sexual abuse or exploitation, or an act or failure to act which presents an imminent risk of serious harm" (Child Abuse Prevention and Treatment Act of 2010, 2010, § 5106g).

Both the WHO and US federal law provide general guidelines for defining the concept of child maltreatment. However, it is up to individual countries and US states to define actual categories or types of maltreatment. For example, neglect is defined by each state in the US based on local standards of care typical to the geographical area or as stated in the state's laws. Standards of care include harm to a child, a parent's ability or intent, a family's access to resources and availability of resources, and community norms (Child Welfare Information Gateway, 2012, para. 10).

Definitions, taken from a variety of resources, are provided in the following chapters in order to give the reader a comprehensive understanding of specific types of maltreatment. Please refer to the laws of your own country or state for the specific definitions that apply in your area.

5   Neglect

Neglect

Neglect is the most often experienced form of child maltreatment (US DHHS, 2013), and it can be the most difficult type of maltreatment to address (DeLong-Hamilton et al., 2015) and identify (McCarroll et al., 2017). Almost 80% of the nearly 700,000 child victims of maltreatment in the US experience child neglect (US DHHS, 2013). More children die annually from neglect than from any other type of maltreatment (US DHHS, Children's Bureau, 2011). In addition, children who die from neglect tend to be below the age of seven (US Government Accountability Office, 2011). Chronic physical neglect or medical neglect are the most common reasons children die (Grayson, 2001). Deaths due to neglect are often hard to investigate and prove because of "lack of definitive evidence, limited investigative and training resources, and differing interpretation of child maltreatment definitions" (US Government Accountability Office, 2011). Children removed from their homes for neglect are less likely to reunify with their families (Bundy-Fazioli et al., 2009). They also experience more days in out-of-home care than children suffering from other types of maltreatment. Because of their complexity and difficulty, neglect cases are often triaged to the bottom of a social worker's caseload (DeLong Hamilton & Bundy-Fazioli, 2013). However, at the same time, because of the complexity and the risk to children, neglect cases need the most attention from social workers.

Definition of Neglect

The Center for Disease Control (CDC) defines neglect as an act of omission:

> Acts of omission are the failure to provide for a child's basic physical, emotional, or educational needs or to protect a child from harm or potential harm. Like acts of commission, harm to a child might not be the intended consequence. The following types of maltreatment

involve acts of omission: physical neglect, emotional neglect, medical and dental neglect, educational neglect, inadequate supervision, and exposure to violent environments.

(CDC, 2016, para. 3)

Neglect is lack of adequate care, such as a lack of food, clothing, medical care, or supervision.

Each state in the US defines neglect differently through state law. In addition, agencies within each state and workers within state agencies use training and experience to further determine what acts or omissions constitute neglect. The lack of a clear definition of neglect across all levels of intervention leads to "inconsistencies in policies, practice, and research" (DePanfilis, 2006, p. 9). Does an elementary school teacher make an abuse report about a student's unkempt appearance and body odor, or does she chalk it up to poor parenting? Does a child protective services worker triage neglect cases to the bottom of the caseload and, instead, focus on the sexual abuse or physical abuse cases because the worker feels the child is not at immediate risk for harm? Does a judge dismiss a case of neglect in court because she does not have a clear understanding of what neglect looks like or how detrimental it can be to a child?

Keep in mind, each country, each state within the US, each agency, and every individual working with children or families may have a slightly different idea about or definition of what constitutes neglect. The following sections provide general definitions for specific types of neglect and case examples of each. It is up to the reader to ensure familiarity with specific definitions or laws related to neglect in her/his individual community.

Physical Neglect

There are several ways in which physical neglect can occur. In each, the child can experience a physical consequence. Physical neglect is broadly defined as "abandoning the child or refusing to accept custody; not providing for basic needs like nutrition, hygiene, or appropriate clothing" (Child Welfare Information Gateway, 2012, para. 12). Physical neglect can occur when a parent or caregiver fails to provide adequate nutrition or clothing to a child, does not address or maintain the hygiene of the child, or does nothing about visible hazards in the home. Physical neglect can also include other forms of reckless disregard of the child's safety and welfare. For example, driving with a child while intoxicated or leaving a young child in a car unattended.

Although physical neglect is defined in terms of a failure to provide for a child's basic needs, it does not mean a family in poverty is necessarily neglectful. A comprehensive assessment of the family can rule out neglect in situations of poverty. In a case where poverty is the main factor making a family unable to meet a child's basic needs, services to alleviate the conditions caused by poverty should be provided to the family rather than intervention by child protective services (CPS). In many states, the CPS worker may ask the parent to volunteer to be under the supervision of the child welfare agency. A parent can refuse supervision. However, if the parent elects voluntary supervision, a worker may be assigned to monitor and offer services to the family as needed, but without court involvement.

Inadequate Supervision

Inadequate supervision can be a category of its own or fall under physical neglect. The general definition of inadequate supervision is, "leaving the child unsupervised (depending on length of time and the child's age and maturity); not protecting the child from safety hazards, providing inadequate caregivers, or engaging in harmful behaviors" (Child Welfare Information Gateway, 2012, para. 12).

There is no universal age at which a child can be left unsupervised or a maximum length of time that a child can be left alone. Fewer than one third of states provide a minimum age at which a child can be left unattended. Where minimum age provisions exist, they are for advisory purposes and are not hard and fast rules. It is important to consider not just the age of the child, but also individual maturity and ability to respond to hazards that may present during a period without supervision. There are some ages for which it would be hard to say any child should be left unsupervised. But due to vast differences in the abilities and maturity of individual children and the spectrum of hazards that may present in any particular home, it is more valuable to evaluate parents' own assessment of the child and the parents' motives for leaving the child unsupervised, rather than jumping to an assumption that a child is inadequately supervised.

Abandonment

Abandonment occurs when a parent deserts the child without arranging for reasonable care and supervision. For example, leaving a child at daycare or with a relative or neighbor and not coming back. This could be hours after a daycare facility closes, a day, or even longer. Typically, daycare facilities file a report if they cannot contact a parent. CPS will intervene and continue to track down the parent. If a parent cannot be found, alternative placement for the child will be found. However, when children are left in the care of a relative, more often than not, the relative will continue to care for the child without CPS involvement. CPS becomes involved in this type of case when the relative finally makes a voluntary or involuntarily report, can no longer financially care for the child, or needs to make an education or health care decision but cannot because they are not a designated legal guardian.

Another form of abandonment involves the refusal to take custody of a child or expulsion of a child from the home. Scenarios might involve a parent refusing to take custody when a child is released from a juvenile justice facility or foster care, or a parent refusing to accept custody of a returned runaway.

Abandonment can also involve expulsion of a child from the home without making adequate arrangements for others to care for the child. This may occur when a parent can no longer manage the behavior of a child or does not like the child's behavior or decision-making.

Educational Neglect

A common type of neglect often seen in the educational system is educational neglect. Educational neglect is "failing to enroll the child in school or homeschool; ignoring special needs: permitting chronic truancy" (Child Welfare Information Gateway, 2012, para. 12).

Each state in the US has specific laws related to compulsory school attendance. If a parent does not enroll a child into an approved educational program (public or private school or appropriate home-schooling plan) by a certain age or soon after relocating, the parent could be cited with educational neglect. Other attendance issues can result in a charge of educational neglect, such as a child missing an extended period of school without notice (typically one month or more) or parents keeping a school-aged child home without valid reasons.

Additionally, when a parent or caregiver permits habitual absenteeism (typically averaging at least five missed school days a month), and after being informed of the situation the parent does not correct the behavior, it could be considered chronic truancy, another form of educational neglect. Some states have laws related to chronic truancy. Not only does CPS become involved in these cases, the parent could be jailed, fined, or experience other sanctions as well.

Inattention to special education needs may also constitute educational neglect. It could include the refusal to allow or the failure to obtain recommended remedial education services, neglect in obtaining or following through with treatment for a child's diagnosed learning disorder, or failure to address or comply with other special education needs or recommendations. However, if the parent can provide a reasonable explanation for the refusal or noncompliance, such as providing alternative services or citing religious or medical reasons, the family may be exempt from a charge of educational neglect.

Emotional Neglect

Emotional neglect is a common type of neglect that is often linked with physical and/or sexual abuse. Emotional neglect is defined as, "isolating the child; not providing affection or emotional support; exposing the child to domestic violence or substance abuse" (Child Welfare Information

Gateway, 2012, para. 12). Emotional neglect is also known as psychological neglect or mental neglect. It can take many forms. Other types of emotional maltreatment include "encouragement or permission of other maladaptive behavior", such as assault, under circumstances "where the parent or caregiver has reason to be aware of the existence and seriousness of the problem but does not intervene" (DePanfilis, 2006, p. 14). Also included in this category is encouraging or permitting a child to engage in drug or alcohol use (DePanfilis, 2006). In such a case, by allowing the child to engage in risky behavior, the parent is not meeting the obligation to protect the child from imminent harm to their emotional condition, which may result from such behavior. Emotional neglect is generally considered the form of maltreatment which is the most difficult to prove.

Inadequate Nurturing or Affection

Inadequate nurturing or affection occurs when a child's basic need for affection, attention, or emotional support are not met on a consistent basis (DePanfilis, 2006). It can occur at any age during childhood, including infancy. Babies need consistent attention from a primary caregiver—someone to hold, cuddle, talk, soothe, provide nourishment, and keep the baby clean and comfortable. These basic acts satisfy the child's need for attachment and are necessary for survival and typical development (Perry, 2001a). When a primary caregiver is not available to meet a child's basic needs or the needs are met inconsistently, the child can experience profound effects that last a lifetime. It can "take many years of hard work to help repair the damage from only a few months of neglect in infancy" (Perry, 2001a, p. 4).

Exposure to Domestic Violence

Exposure to Domestic Violence occurs when a child is present during chronic or extreme partner abuse (DePanfilis, 2006). Although it may be self-explanatory, exposure to domestic violence can occur in a variety of ways: a child could be in another room but hear a violent episode occurring, a child could be in the same room and observe a violent act occurring, or a child could be placed in harm's way and suffer injuries as a result of a violent episode. In the latter case, a parent might be cited for child physical abuse as well as emotional abuse.

As domestic violence became a socially recognized problem and exposure to domestic violence was identified as a form of neglect, mothers, who are more often victims of the violence, were more likely to be the alleged perpetrators of this form of neglect, not the abusers themselves. A New York State Court of Appeals decision in a class-action lawsuit in New York City helped clarify when it is appropriate for child protection services to charge a domestic violence victim as a perpetrator of exposure to domestic violence:

the battered mother is charged with neglect not because she is a victim of domestic violence or because her children witnessed the abuse, but rather because a preponderance of the evidence establishes that the children were actually or imminently harmed by reason of her failure to exercise even minimal care in providing them with proper oversight.

(*Nicholson v. Scoppetta*, 2004, NY Slip Op 07617, 3 NY3d 257)

The court in *Nicholson v. Scoppetta* also provided guidance on removing children from a victim parent. If there are mechanisms through which the victim parent, even with the assistance of the child protective services system, can mitigate the child's exposure to violence while remaining together, then the child should not be removed from the victim parent.

Medical Neglect

Medical neglect is defined as "delaying or denying recommended health care for the child" (Child Welfare Information Gateway, 2012, para. 12). The Child Abuse Prevention and Treatment Act of 2010 (2010) defines medical neglect as the "withholding of medically indicated treatment" that a physician may deem "reasonable" or "effective in ameliorating or correcting all such conditions." The refusal of health care and a delay in health care for a child are included in the category of medical neglect.

A family may be protected from a charge of medical neglect due to a constitutionally protected right to practice religious beliefs. Families with a specific religious belief regarding medical care cannot be held accountable if harm occurs to a child because of such a belief. However, the government, through their *parens patriae* authority (see Chapter 2) can step in and require the child receive medical care in opposition to a family's religious beliefs. The state would need to show that failure to provide the care would cause harm to the child.

Refusal of Health Care

Refusal of health care occurs when a parent or caregiver fails to provide or allow needed care in accordance with the recommendations of a "competent health care professional, for a physical injury, illness, medical condition, or impairment" (DePanfilis, 2006, p. 12). A good example of refusal of health care is when a parent refuses to obtain an x-ray for an injury after a health care professional indicates a child may have a broken bone.

Delay in Health Care

Delay in health care occurs when a parent or caregiver fails "to seek timely and appropriate medical care for a serious health problem that any reasonable person would have recognized as needing professional medical attention" (DePanfilis, 2006, p. 12). For example, if a toddler falls and suffers a laceration that needs stitches, and a parent or caregiver does not take the child for appropriate medical treatment, then it is an instance of delay in health care. The problem can be compounded if a wound becomes infected or the child suffers further effects or illness based on the parent's refusal to seek care.

Consequences of Neglect

While the impact of neglect on a child may be less visible than the effects of physical or sexual abuse, the consequences of neglect can be worse and longer lasting than other types of maltreatment. All areas of a child's development can be affected by neglect, including health, physical development, intellectual and cognitive development, emotional and psychological development, and social and behavioral development (DePanfilis, 2006; Perry, 2001a; Perry & Pollard, 1997). The consequences of neglect are influenced by other factors, such as the child's age; the presence of protective factors; the frequency, duration, and severity of neglect; and the relationship between the child and parent or caregiver (DePanfilis, 2006; Chalk et al., 2002).

Neglect experienced by a young child can actually alter the physical growth and organization of the brain (Perry & Pollard, 1997). During the first three years of life, the brain grows faster than at any other time. Therefore, children neglected early in life may exhibit a spectrum of problems after the neglect and into later childhood and adulthood (Perry, 2001a).

Children who have been neglected at any point in time may experience developmental delays in language, social behaviors, and cognitive development (Perry, 2001a). They may exhibit odd eating behaviors, such as hoarding, hiding, or binging on food. Children who have experienced neglect may engage in problematic self-soothing behaviors, such as head banging, rocking, or self-injury (i.e., scratching, biting, cutting). Additionally, emotional and mental health problems stemming from childhood neglect, such as depression and anxiety, are common (Perry, 2001a).

Health and Physical Development of a Child

Neglect can cause physical impairments in children, such as failure to thrive in infants, compromised health, malnourishment, and stunted physical growth. Researchers found that children neglected in early life have noticeably smaller frames and less brain growth (DeBellis, 2005; Perry, 2001a). They also may experience hyperarousal, they may be on constant guard against threats, or they may disassociate as a coping mechanism (Johnson-Reid et al., 2004; Perry 1996; Perry, 2001b). Neglected children are often labeled daydreamers, because they zone out when they feel threatened (Perry & Szalavitz, 2006). In addition, research indicates that experiencing neglect along with other forms of maltreatment worsens the impact of the maltreatment (Smith & Fong, 2004).

Intellectual and Cognitive Development

Child victims of neglect often have lower IQs, poor academic performance, and delayed or impaired language development (DePanfilis, 2006; Shonkoff & Phillips, 2000). These delays affect all aspects of the child's life, including relationships with family and peers, academic progress, and social and emotional well-being.

Emotional and psychological development

Neglect has been linked to deficiencies in child self-esteem, attachment, and trust (DePanfilis, 2006; Ludy-Dobson & Perry, 2010). Children who suffer trauma are often diagnosed with PTSD, depression, disassociation, and conduct disorders (Ludy-Dobson & Perry, 2010). These mental health issues often persist into adulthood. Other researchers have linked neglect to the diagnosis of personality disorders in adulthood (DePanfilis, 2006) and studied the relationship between childhood trauma and psychosis (Read et al., 2014).

Social and Behavioral Development

Neglect can lead to interpersonal relationship problems, aggression, and conduct disorders (DePanfilis, 2006). Research has found a tie between neglect and increased illegal behavior, running away from home, substance abuse in adulthood and PTSD symptoms from childhood into adulthood (DePanfilis, 2006; Ludy-Dobson & Perry, 2010; Milot et al., 2010). Other types of behavioral issues are also associated with trauma including antisocial behaviors and engagement in high-risk sexual behavior and teenage pregnancy (Ludy-Dobson & Perry, 2010).

Risk and Protective Factors for Neglect

Risk and protective factors are those factors that put a child at risk for neglect or provide a defense from neglect. Risk and protective factors derive from the micro, mezzo, and macro areas of a child's environment.

Risk factors are attributes, characteristics, or exposures that increase the likelihood that a particular individual will experience a given condition (WHO, 2016). In the case of neglect, risk factors are attributes, characteristics, or conditions to which a child or family might be exposed that statistically increase the likelihood that a child will be neglected. Keep in mind, however, these are risk factors, and they do not cause neglect. Instead, experiences due to the presence of risk factors are thought to increase the stress level in a family, which can lead to neglect. Just because a child or family exhibits or experiences one or more risk factors does not mean that a child will definitively experience neglect.

Protective factors are the opposite of risk factors. The presence of protective factors increases the likelihood of positive outcomes and lessens the likelihood of negative consequences from exposures to risk (WHO, 2016). In short, risk is mitigated by protective factors.

Due to the complex relationship between risk and protective factors, a comprehensive assessment of the family is important and necessary to determine if a child is at risk for neglect and the extent of risk. It is essential to look at all of the factors, both risk and protective, to get a complete picture of a child's level of risk.

At the individual level, a child's characteristics, such as physical appearance, behavior, or disability, can place a child at risk for neglect. At a micro level, very important factors to consider when completing a risk assessment include child (age or developmental delays), parent, or family characteristics (parent age, socioeconomic status, health, mental health, substance abuse); poverty; domestic violence; stress levels; and the home environment (Bundy-Fazioli & DeLong-Hamilton, 2010; DePanfilis, 2006). At the mezzo level, risk and protective factor considerations include the surrounding environment, such as neighborhood, community, school and other local systems (i.e., unsafe neighborhoods, community acceptance of neglect, environmental hazards) (Bundy-Fazioli & DeLong-Hamilton, 2010; Cash & Wilke, 2003; DePanfilis, 2006). Lastly, at the macro level, state or country laws, the child protective system, or the lack of a child protective system can also be either risk or protective factors (Bundy-Fazioli & DeLong-Hamilton, 2010).

Protective factors play a large part in reducing the chance of neglect. In families where one or more of the following factors have been found, children are less likely to experience neglect: nurturing parents with a strong parent-child attachment, parental knowledge of parenting skills and child development, parental resilience, social connections, concrete forms of support, or children with social and emotional competence (Bundy-Fazioli & DeLong-Hamilton, 2010; DePanfilis, 2006).

Family Characteristics

There are family characteristics associated with neglectful behavior toward children. Family risk factors include marital problems, domestic violence, single-parenthood, family composition, unemployment, financial stress, and parent characteristics (DePanfilis, 2006).

Stress

Families who neglect their children are more likely to experience higher stress than other families. Stress can come from financial difficulties, substance abuse problems, housing problems, illness, or other problems (DePanfilis, 2006). Additional stress within a family can increase emotions, and a parent may find it difficult to manage, which can lead to neglect (Goldman & Salus, 2003).

Communication

Family communication and interaction patterns can contribute to the risk of neglect. Negative interaction patterns can include expressions of negative emotions, a lack of empathy, the lack of emotional closeness, poor negotiation skills, or an unwillingness to take responsibility for actions (Connell-Carrick, 2003). There may also be less engagement between the parent and child in families that experience neglect (Dubowitz & Black, 2001; Goldman & Salus, 2003).

Violence

Domestic violence also increases the likelihood of neglect (Antle et al., 2007; Bragg, 2003; Shepard & Raschick, 1999). Even if a child is not physically injured, perpetrators of domestic violence can be found responsible for neglect or, potentially, physical abuse. Children in the proximity of a violent encounter may be at risk of physical injury. Witnessing domestic violence may harm a child's emotional or mental condition as well. Additionally, victims of domestic violence have been found to have failed to protect their children from harm because they were unable or unwilling to engage with the violent partner in order to safeguard the child (Lemon, 1999).

Support

Social support is another important consideration. Inefficient social networks or difficulties in finding childcare can put children at risk for neglect, especially in families with parental substance abuse issues (Cash & Wilke, 2003).

Family Composition

Single parent families have a higher risk of neglect (Connell-Carrick, 2003). Larger families also have an increased risk (Dubowitz, et al., 2011). Limited time and money are the primary factors that influence risk in single parent and large families. Single parents must juggle running a household, working, and raising children. Because the responsibility falls on one person, the parent may lack availability to supervise and spend time with a child, which may lead to neglect (DePanfilis, 2006). Additionally, many single parents live close to or below the poverty line.

Parent Characteristics

There are several parent characteristics that increase the likelihood that children will be neglected.

Childhood Victimization

Parents who were maltreated as children are more likely to neglect their own children (Connell-Carrick, 2003; Renner & Slack, 2006). Mothers who experienced sexual abuse are three times more likely to neglect their children (Zuravin & DiBlasio, 1996). Other related characteristics have also been found to increase the risk of neglect, such as a history of running away and/or placement in foster care (Gershater-Molko & Lutzker, 1999) and growing up in an unstable or hostile home (Gaudin, 1993).

Cognitive Functioning

Cognitive functioning also plays a role in neglectful family dynamics. Parents with poor problem-solving skills, poor parenting skills, or inadequate knowledge of child development are at higher risk of engaging in neglectful behavior with their children (Dubowitz & Black, 2001).

Personality Characteristics

There are also specific parental personality characteristics linked to the neglect of children. Parents who had insecure attachments to or poor relationships with their own parents are at greater risk of engaging in neglectful behavior (Thomlison, 1997). Additionally, poor coping skills, social incompetence, or an inability to come to terms with a history of maltreatment can increase the chance of neglect in a family (Thomlison, 1997). Many times, parents do not recognize that their behaviors were neglectful (Coohey, 2003).

Substance Abuse

Substance abuse plays a large role in child neglect. In fact, the majority of neglect reports relate to parental substance abuse. Parents who abuse alcohol or other drugs are more likely to neglect their children (Carter & Myers, 2007; Dubowitz et al., 2011; Goldman & Salus, 2003; Lee, 2012; Ondersma, 2002). When the parent is impaired due to the use or abuse of substances, they may not make appropriate decisions (DePanfilis, 2006). In addition, a parent experiencing substance abuse may put their own needs ahead of children's needs and may spend money on substances rather than on basic necessities needed to care for children.

Mental Health

Many researchers have linked depression and anxiety to the neglect of children. Both maternal (Lee, 2012; Mustillo et al., 2011; Perry, 2001a) and paternal depression (Dubowitz et al., 2011; Epkins & Harper, 2016; Lee et al., 2012) have been found to be significant risk factors for neglectful parenting.

Child Characteristics

Some of the most important factors that increase the risk of neglect are the specific characteristics of the child. Although children of all ages can experience neglect, the risk declines as a child ages (Child Welfare Information Gateway, 2012; DePanfilis, 2006). Child neglect can be more detrimental to children ages three and younger, because they are the most vulnerable, and the most damage can be done during the ages when the brain is still developing (Ludy-Dobson & Perry, 2010; Perry, 2001a; Perry & Pollard, 1997).

Research has found that, when it comes to neglect, there is very little difference between male and female children. Generally, boys and girls are at equal risk of experiencing this form of maltreatment (US DHHS, 2016). However, research confirms that the prevalence of neglect differs by race. Black children are more likely to be found victims of neglect than children of other races (US DHHS, 2010). Further studies show, however, that race itself is not the actual risk factor. Rather, there is an increased likelihood that Black children live in poverty, and they are at a higher risk of neglect due to the stresses of the family's financial condition (Johnson-Reid et al., 2013). In addition, children with mental or physical disabilities are also at greater risk compared to children without disabilities (ACF, 2012).

Temperament and Behavior

Children prone to exhibiting irritable behavior or those that are difficult to soothe are at higher risk of neglect (Harrington et al., 1998). The added stress of caring for an irritable child can strain the parent-child relationship, often leading to emotional neglect. Child protective services workers who focus on "difficult" children may overlook child victims of neglect who rarely act out. These children may be withdrawn, passive, or nonassertive (DePanfilis, 2006; Sherman & Holden, 2000).

Special Needs

Children who have special needs or disabilities are more likely to be neglected than children who do not (Crosse et al., n.d.; Goldman & Salus, 2003). Like young children, this population is more vulnerable and typically needs more care, which places additional stress on a parent or caregiver.

Additional parental stress and the need for more care create a greater risk for neglect (Kolko, 2002; Zipper & Simeonsson, 1997).

Assessment of Neglect

Often neglect is triaged to the bottom of the list behind other types of maltreatment (Bundy-Fazioli & DeLong-Hamilton, 2013). However, taking the time to complete a comprehensive assessment of neglect cases and provide the appropriate interventions as soon as possible can prevent neglect from becoming chronic and acute.

A key factor in a risk assessment for neglect is looking at previous incidents of neglect or a pattern of neglect. Discerning a pattern of neglect can provide the child welfare worker a picture of what has occurred over time and assist in determining services for the family (DePanfilis, 2006).

When preparing for and conducting an assessment of neglect, the child welfare worker should use basic social work skills to develop a relationship and trust with the parent. This can include the way questions are asked during the assessment process and consideration of cultural practices or beliefs (DePanfilis, 2006). A trusting relationship increases the likelihood that a case plan will be successfully completed (Bundy-Fazioli, 2009).

Because neglect is complex, it is most often described, defined, and assessed using a socio-ecological perspective, which considers all factors that could contribute to the neglect (Dubowitz et al., 2005), including societal and environmental factors (Erikson & Egeland, 2002). A multi-dimensional, ecological-systems-perspective framework for assessment should focus on the interdependency of individuals within their environment (Bundy-Fazioli & DeLong-Hamilton, 2010; Payne, 2014). The Bundy-Fazioli and DeLong Hamilton (2010) multi-dimensional framework for assessment is based on ecological systems theory. This model takes into consideration all systems in which a family exists and interacts (Payne, 2014). The model provides a guideline for child welfare workers to identify family strengths and challenges from a parental perspective. The assessment encourages discussion and communication between social worker and parent, which promotes a healthy working relationship between the two. The model has three focus areas: (1) child and family strengths and challenges, (2) parental perception and awareness, and (3) agency involvement (Bundy-Fazioli & DeLong-Hamilton, 2010) (Table 5.1).

Model Assessment

Focus 1: Child and Family Strengths and Challenges

The assessment process starts with gathering a thorough history of the child and parent. Because parents tend to parent children in the same manner as they were parented, it is important to explore how a child was previously

Table 5.1 Multi-Dimensional Framework for Assessment ★PC=parental control

Areas of Strengths & Challenges	Parents' Perception and Awareness			Agency Involvement	
	History Pattern	Change beyond PC★	Change within PC★	Current	Past

Parent History

Significant Events

Child History

Developmental Milestones

Parent Well-being

- Mental health status
- Substance use & abuse
- Domestic violence
- Trauma, grief, loss
- Communication skills
- Physical health
- Education learning

Child Well-being

- Mental health status
- Substance use & abuse
- Type of neglect/abuse
- Trauma, grief, loss
- Friends & activities
- Physical health
- Education learning

Parent-Child/Family Well-being

- Familial status (who lives in the home?)
- Basic needs (housing, food, clothes)
- Parenting skills (discipline, attachment, safety, basic needs, protection, values)
- Parent-child interaction
- Child interaction with relatives

Community/ Environmental

- Housing
- Neighborhood

(continued)

Areas of Strengths & Challenges	Parents' Perception and Awareness			Agency Involvement	
	History Pattern	Change beyond PC★	Change within PC★	Current	Past
■ Child/family activities (church, school, etc)					
■ Transportation					
Social Supports					
■ Friends					
■ Family					
■ Job					
Financial Supports					
■ Employment					

and is currently being cared for (Perry & Szalavitz, 2006). When gathering the child's history, it is important to find out when developmental milestones were met as the information can assist in discovering the extent that development may have been disrupted by the neglect (Perry & Szalavitz, 2006). While exploring the family history, social workers should list all strengths and challenges that the family is currently experiencing or may have experienced in the past. During the assessment process, observation of parent-child interaction can also be helpful and provide information about the type of relationship that has developed (Bowlby, 2005, pp. 137–57).

Categories in the first section of the model assessment are well-being, community/environment, social support, and financial support.

Focus 2: Parental Perceptions and Awareness

More often than not, the parent's perception of the problem is quite different from the child welfare worker's perception. In many neglect cases, parents are often struggling with multiple problems that they feel are beyond their control (Bundy-Fazioli & DeLong-Hamilton, 2010). Information about the parent's view can guide the child welfare worker and assist with making recommendations for interventions.

Focus 3: Agency Involvement

Often families involved in the child welfare system are also involved with numerous other service providers. Obtaining a history of a family's service providers and details about those services that were helpful or those that were not can provide valuable information that allows the child welfare worker to be more responsive and plan for appropriate interventions

(Bundy-Fazioli & DeLong-Hamilton, 2010). An approach that takes other services into account will help the family successfully complete a case plan instead of making them feel bogged down with additional or excessive mandated tasks, which can lead to non-compliance with a case plan or court order.

As well as completing a comprehensive multi-dimensional assessment, child welfare workers should also determine the severity of the neglect and the risk of future harm.

Classifying Neglect

Child welfare workers should ask two questions: Do the conditions or circumstances indicate that a child's basic needs are unmet? and What harm or threat of harm may have resulted? (DePanfilis, 2006, p. 46). The answers to these two questions can assist the child welfare worker in determining the degree or level of harm the child may have suffered and whether or not there may be risk for future harm.

Unlike physical abuse or sexual abuse, neglect can be classified into three types.

Mild Neglect

Mild neglect cases are acts of omission that typically do not require CPS to open a case but might require some type of intervention (DePanfilis, 2006). For example, after a toddler is treated in an emergency room for a laceration sustained while playing alone outside, a parent may need educational information about the importance of supervision.

Moderate Neglect

Moderate neglect cases happen when an intervention does not work or if a child is moderately harmed (DePanfilis, 2006). For example, the toddler referenced above continues to play alone outside without supervision and is treated again for another injury. At this point, CPS would be concerned with the parents' failure to respond to recommendations.

Severe Neglect

Severe neglect cases typically involve long-term neglect that causes harm to a child (DePanfilis, 2006). For example, a parent with a substance abuse issue goes out on a binge and leaves a young child alone for a significant length of time with no supervision. At this point, CPS would become involved and open an official case in order to intervene with the family to ensure the child has appropriate supervision and the parent receives help.

Chronic Neglect

Assessing for neglect not only entails classifying neglect, it also considers the length of time the neglect has occurred. CPS workers should look for patterns of neglect, including previous reports of neglect, and consider how past reports were finalized (e.g., unfounded, founded, etc.). Although a current allegation of neglect alone may not be enough to open a child welfare case, a history of allegations may establish a pattern that provides justification for CPS intervention.

Chronic neglect is defined as "an ongoing, serious pattern of deprivation of a child's basic physical, developmental, and emotional needs by a parent or caregiver that results in accumulation of harm to the child" (Gilmore & Kaplan, 2009, slide 8). Zuravin (2001) describes chronicity as "patterns of the same acts or omissions that extend over time or recur over time" (p. 50).

Risk of Future Neglect

An assessment of neglect should also include an evaluation of the risk of future neglect. Each state's child protective services agency utilizes evidence-based assessment tools designed to determine the risk of future neglect in a family. These tools are designed to help practitioners decide whether intervention with the family is necessary and, if so, what type of intervention should take place. Consult your local child protective services agencies for the latest tools they are using in the field.

Treatment of Neglect

Families with a history of neglect need "quick engagement and effective treatments" (Dawson & Berry, 2002, p. 305). If appropriate intervention is not received in a timely manner, the children of these families are more likely to experience unstable environments and long-lasting deleterious effects to their well-being.

Initially, it is important to minimize any immediate risk to the child. Once risk is identified, targeted services or resources can be implemented.

DePanfilis (2006) offers six steps for effective intervention:

1   Building a relationship with the family,
2   Developing a case and safety plan,
3   Establishing concrete goals,
4   Targeting outcomes,
5   Tracking family progress, and
6   Analyzing and evaluating family progress.

There are a variety of interventions that can be employed when working with families who neglect. The intervention depends on the type of neglect, the circumstances of the family, and the age of the child. Child-centered interventions include daycare or educationally based services, medical care, mentoring, or behavioral or emotional treatment (DePanfilis, 2006). Parent-centered interventions include programs to improve parenting skills and the parent-child relationship, mental health treatment programs, substance abuse treatment programs, and programs that address domestic violence (DePanfilis, 2006). Family-centered interventions involve parents and children. Typically, they also include coordination of multiple providers, faith-based programs, and community-based programs. Some of these services could include training or education about child development, behavioral and social skills, and how to improve relationships (DePanfilis, 2006). Concrete resources obtained from social supports, community services, and faith-based programs are also helpful for families with a history of neglect. Concrete services and resources can reduce stress on the family, thereby reducing the risk of neglect. Other interventions specifically targeted at parents include cognitive-behavioral programs, such as home safety; affective skills training; and initiatives to help stimulate infant development (DePanfilis, 2006). While the preferred intervention into any family aims to keep the family intact, out-of-home placement, including foster care, may be appropriate in some cases of neglect.

Change is difficult. If the family is not ready or prepared to begin making change, even the most effective intervention will fail. During any intervention process, it is important to keep the stages of the change model in mind (Chang et al., 2009).

Case Examples and Questions

For each of the case examples, please answer the following questions:

1   Which type(s) of neglect may be involved in this case?
2   What risk and protective factors related to family, child, and parent characteristics seem to be relevant in this case?
3   What does the parent's awareness seem to be of the important issues identified?
4   Is there prior involvement with the child welfare system?

    (A)   And, if so, how does it impact your assessment of the case?

5   Do you think neglect is occurring?

    (A)   And, if so, how would you classify the neglect you think is occurring (mild, moderate, severe, chronic)?

6   What intervention(s) do you think should be provided to the family? Why?

Case One: Inadequate Supervision

Ms. Jones has two children: a 6-year-old and an 8-year-old. She is a single mom who works in a minimum-, hourly-wage job. She has no benefits, such as health insurance or sick leave. She relies on Medicaid for her children's health care, but she does not have health insurance herself. She never married the father of her children, and he has not been present in the children's lives for several years. Ms. Jones does not know where the father is and does not receive child support. The 6-year-old attends kindergarten. The 8-year-old attends third grade in the local public school. Both children are doing well in school and have met developmental milestones for their ages. Although finances are very tight, the family is functioning well. One day, the 8-year-old child wakes with a fever. Ms. Jones makes the decision to leave the sick child home alone so she can go to work. If Ms. Jones were to miss work to stay home with her child, she would lose pay for the day, and the rest of her hours for the week might be cut as well. In order to pay her bills and support her children, she must go to work. The morning is uneventful, and the child sleeps soundly. At lunchtime, the child decides he is feeling better and attempts to make macaroni and cheese in the microwave (his mother said not to use the stove). The food is cooked too long and creates a strong burnt smell, which goes into the apartment hallway. One of the neighbors, who happens to be walking by, smells the odor and becomes concerned. She calls the apartment manager, who goes to the Jones apartment to check on the situation. The child opens the door when the manager knocks. The manager asks to speak to his mother. When the child replies that his mother is not home, the manager asks if everything is ok, then tells the child to close and lock the door and not leave the apartment. The manager calls child protective services to make a report. Ms. Jones is now under investigation for inadequate supervision.

Case Two: Medical Neglect

Jane is a 14-year-old girl who has suffered with an unknown, serious medical condition for the past two years. Jane's parents are married and have a stable relationship. The marriage is a traditional one. The father works, and the mother stays home to care for the children and the home. Jane is the youngest of five children in the family. Jane's family has religious beliefs that prohibit medical intervention of any sort. Instead, they rely on natural remedies and prayer. Although Jane and her parents have been able to manage her medical condition for the past two years, Jane is beginning to have symptoms that create pain and discomfort. In fact, recently Jane had such severe pain that her mother took her to an urgent care center, where the physician recommended hospitalization and surgery. Because the family does not believe in traditional medical intervention, the mother declined, took Jane home, and told Jane not to mention the urgent care visit to anyone. Two days later, after the father leaves for work and the rest of the children leave for school, the mother goes into Jane's room to check on her. Jane is non-responsive, and her breathing is shallow. The mother tries to revive her with no result. She calls 911, and Jane is rushed in an ambulance to the hospital. An examination by an emergency physician determines that Jane is in very critical condition, which could have been averted if her mother had admitted her to the hospital after the urgent care visit. The physician calls child protective services, and the family is now under investigation. Jane remains in the hospital in the intensive care unit.

Case Three: Failure to Thrive

Kelly is an 18-year-old mother. She gave birth to her son, Kody, while living with her parents. Since that time, she graduated from high school and obtained a part-time job as a receptionist. She and Kody's father, Justin, married when Kody was six months old, and they all live in a small apartment together. Justin is 21 years old and works 60 hours a week as a mechanic. Kelly and Justin fight quite a bit. The fighting consists of yelling and has not escalated to physical violence. However, the fights occur several times a week. They typically end with Justin storming out of the apartment and Kelly crying. The couple has difficulty communicating their needs. When they fight, Kody is often in the room. Kody attends daycare while Kelly is at work. He is typically at the center in the mornings, five days a week. Every six months Kody's daycare provider is required to complete an assessment on each child in her class. While completing Kody's assessment, the daycare provider realizes he is very behind the other 1-year-olds in the class. The provider had previously noted Kody's lagging development, but didn't realize how far behind he was until she completed the assessment. Typically, most 1-year-old children walk and use a small vocabulary of words. Kody does not talk at all, and he is not walking yet. When his mother drops him off, he usually stays in the same spot most of the morning and plays with whatever toy is nearby. He does not fuss or cry and appears content. Kody is also small for his age and does not have a lot of body fat. Compared to the other children in the class, he is much smaller and appears to be younger. At lunchtime it is difficult to get him to eat and drink. Recently, Kody came to daycare with bruises on his legs and arms. Kelly told the daycare provider that Kody had been attempting to walk but had fallen down a lot. The provider, concerned about Kody based on the assessment and bruises, makes a report to child protective services.

References

ACF (Administration for Children and Families). (2012). *Child Maltreatment: 2011 Report*. Washington, DC: US Department of Health and Human Services.

Antle, B.F., Barbee, A.P., Sullivan, D., Yankeelov, P., Johnson, L., & Cunningham, M.R. (2007). The Relationship between Domestic Violence and Child Neglect. *Brief Treatment and Crisis Intervention*, 7 (4), 364–382.

Bowlby, J. (2005). *A Secure Base: Parent-Child Attachment and Healthy Human Development*. London: Routledge.

Bragg, H.L. (2003). Child Protection in Families Experiencing Domestic Violence. *Child Welfare Information Gateway.* Retrieved from: http://www.childwelfare. gov/pubs/usermanuals/domesticviolence/domesticviolence.pdf.

Bundy-Fazioli, K. (2009). A Qualitative Examination of Power between Child Welfare Workers and Parents. *British Journal of Social Work*, 39 (8), 1447–1464.

Bundy-Fazioli, K. & DeLong-Hamilton, T. (2010). Educating Social Workers on Child Neglect: A Multi-Dimensional Framework for Assessment. *The International Journal of Continuing Social Work Education*, 13 (1), 40–46.

Bundy-Fazioli, K. & DeLong-Hamilton, T. (2013). A Qualitative Study Exploring Mothers' Perception of Child Neglect. *Children and Youth Services Review*, 34 (3), 250–266.

Bundy-Fazioli, K., Winokur, M., & DeLong-Hamilton, T. (2009). Placement Outcomes for Children Removed for Neglect Compared to Children Removed for Abuse. *Child Welfare*, 88 (3), 85–102.

Carter, V. & Myers, M.R. (2007). Exploring the Risks of Substantiated Physical Neglect Related to Poverty and Parental Characteristics: A National Sample. *Children and Youth Services Review*, 29 (1), 110–121.

Cash, S.J. & Wilke, D.J. (2003). An Ecological Model of Maternal Substance Abuse and Child Neglect: Issues, Analysis, and Recommendations. *American Journal of Orthopsychiatry*, 73 (4), 392–404.

CDC (Centers for Disease Control). (2016). Child Abuse and Neglect Definitions. *CDC: Centers for Disease Control and Prevention.* Retrieved from: http://www.cdc. gov/ViolencePrevention/childmaltreatment/definitions.html.

Chalk, R., Gibbons, A., & Scarupa, H.J. (2002). The Multiple Dimensions of Child Abuse and Neglect: New Insights into an Old Problem. *Child Trends Research Brief.* Retrieved February 2012 from: http://www.childtrends.org/files/Child AbuseRB.pdf.

Chang, V.N., Scott, S.T., & Decker, C.L. (2009). *Developing Helping Skills: A Step-by-Step Approach.* Belmont, CA: Brooks/Cole Cengage Learning.

Child Abuse Prevention and Treatment Act of 2010. (2010). 42 U.S.C. § 5106g.

Child Welfare Information Gateway. (2012). *Acts of Omission: An Overview of Child Neglect.* Washington, DC: US Department of Health and Human Services, Children's Bureau.

Connell-Carrick, K. (2003). A Critical Review of the Empirical Literature: Identifying Correlates of Child Neglect. *Child and Adolescent Social Work*, 20 (5), 389–425.

Coohey, C. (2003). Making Judgments about Risk in Substantiated Cases of Supervisory Neglect. *Child Abuse and Neglect*, 27 (7), 821–840.

Crosse, S.B., Kaye, E., & Ratnofsky, A.C. (n.d.). *A Report on the Maltreatment of Children with Disabilities.* Washington, DC: US Department of Health and Human Services, NCCAN.

Dawson, K. & Berry, M. (2002). Engaging Families in Child Welfare Services: An Evidence-Based Approach to Best Practice. *Child Welfare League of America*, 71 (2), 293–317.

DeBellis, M.D. (2005). The Psychobiology of Neglect. *Child Maltreatment*, 10, 150–172.

DeLong Hamilton, T. & Bundy-Fazioli, K. (2013). Exploring the Complexities of Child Neglect: Ethical Issues of Child Welfare Practice. *Journal of Social Work Values and Ethics*, 10 (2), 14–24.

DeLong-Hamilton, T., Krase, K., & Bundy-Fazioli, K. (2015). Exploring Child Welfare Workers' Experiences with Neglect Cases: A Qualitative Study. *Journal of Public Child Welfare*, 10 (1), 21–38.

DePanfilis, D. (2006). *Child Neglect: A Guide for Prevention, Assessment, and Intervention*. Washington, DC: US Department of Health and Human Services Administration for Children and Families Administration on Children, Youth and Families Children's Bureau Office on Child Abuse and Neglect.

Dubowitz, H. & Black, M. M. (2001). Child Neglect. In R.M. Reece & S. Ludwig (Eds.), *Child Abuse: Medical Diagnosis and Management*, 2nd edition, 339–362. Philadelphia, PA: Lea & Febiger.

Dubowitz, H., Kim, J., Black, M.M., Weisbart, C., Semiatin, J., Magder, L.S. (2011). Identifying Children at High Risk for a Child Maltreatment Report. *Child Abuse and Neglect*, 35 (2), 96–104.

Dubowitz, H., Newton, R.R., Litrownik, A.J., Lewis, T., Briggs, E.C., Thompson, R., English, D., Lee, L.C., & Feerick, M.M. (2005). Examination of a Conceptual Model of Child Neglect. *Child Maltreatment*, 10 (2), 173–189.

Epkins, C.C. & Harper, S.L. (2016). Mothers' and Fathers' Parental Warmth, Hostility/Rejection/Neglect, and Behavioral Control: Specific and Unique Relations with Parents' Depression vs. Anxiety Symptoms. *Parenting*, 16 (2), 125–145.

Erickson, M.F. & Egeland, B. (2002). Child Neglect. In J. Briere, L. Berliner, C.T. Hendrix, C. Jenny, & T. Reid (Eds.), *The APSAC Handbook on Child Maltreatment*, 2nd edition, 3–20. Thousand Oaks, CA: Sage Publications.

Gaudin, J.M., Jr. (1993). *Child Neglect: A Guide for Intervention (HHS-105-89-1730)*. US Department of Health and Human Services Administration for Children and Families. Washington, DC: Westover Consultants.

Gershater-Molko, R.M. & Lutzker, J. R. (1999). Child Neglect. In R.T. Ammerman & M. Hersen (Eds.), *Assessment of Family Violence: A Clinical and Legal Sourcebook*, 2nd edition, 157–183. New York: John Wiley & Sons.

Gilmore, D. & Kaplan, C. (2009). Chronic Families, Chronic Neglect [PowerPoint slides]. *American Humane Association*. Retrieved February 2012 from: http://www.americanhumane.org/assets/pdfs/children/pc-chronic-families-chronic-neglect.pdf.

Goldman, J. & Salus, M.K. (2003). *A Coordinated Response to Child Abuse and Neglect: The Foundation for Practice*. Washington, DC: US Department of Health and Human Services, Administration for Children and Families, Administration on Children, Youth and Families, Children's Bureau, Office on Child Abuse and Neglect.

Grayson, J. (2001). The State of Child Neglect. In T.D. Morton & B. Salovitz (Eds.), *The CPS Response to Child Neglect: An Administrator's Guide to Theory, Policy, Program Design and Case Practice*, 1–36. Duluth, GA: National Resource Center on Child Maltreatment. Retrieved February 2012 from: http://www.nrccps.org/PDF/CPSResponsetoChildNeglect.pdf.

Harrington, D., Black, M.M., Starr, R.H., & Dubowitz, H. (1998). Child Neglect: Relation to Child Temperament and Family Context. *American Journal of Orthopsychiatry*, 68 (1), 108–116.

Johnson-Reid, M., Drake, B., Kim, J., Porterfield, S., & Han, L. (2004). A Prospective Analysis of the Relationship between Reported Child Maltreatment and Special Education Eligibility among Poor Children. *Child Maltreatment*, 9 (4), 382–394.

Johnson-Reid, M., Drake, B., & Zhou, P. (2013). Neglect Subtypes, Race, and Poverty: Individual, Family, and Service Characteristics. *Child Maltreatment*, 18 (1), 30–41.

Kolko, D.J. (2002). Child Physical Abuse. In J.E.B. Myers, L. Berliner, J. Briere, C.T. Hendrix, C. Jenny, & T.A. Reid (Eds.), *The APSAC Handbook on Child Maltreatment*, 2nd edition, 21–54. Thousand Oaks, CA: Sage.

Lee, S.J. (2012). Parental and Household Characteristics Associated with Child Neglect and Child Protective Services Involvement. *Social Service Research*, 39 (2), 171–187.

Lee, S.J., Taylor, C.A., & Bellamy, J.L. (2012). Paternal Depression and Risk for Child Neglect in Father-Involved Families of Young Children. *Child Abuse and Neglect*, 36 (5), 461–469.

Lemon, N.K.D. (1999). The Legal System's Response to Children Exposed to Domestic Violence. *Future of Children*, 9 (3), 67–83.

Ludy-Dobson, C.R. & Perry, B.D. (2010). The Role of Healthy Relational Interactions in Buffering the Impact of Childhood Trauma. In E. Gil (Ed.), *Working with Children to Heal Interpersonal Trauma: The Power of Play*, 26–43. New York: The Guilford Press.

McCarroll, J.E., Fisher, J.E., Cozza, S.J., Robichaux, R.J., & Fullerton, C.S. (2017). Characteristics, Classification, and Prevention of Child Maltreatment Fatalities. *Military Medicine*, 182 (1), 1551–1557.

Milot, T., St-Laurent, D., Éthier, L.S., & Provost, M.A. (2010). Trauma-Related Symptoms in Neglected Preschoolers and Affective Quality of Mother-Child Communication. *Child Maltreatment*, 15 (4), 293–304.

Mustillo, S.A., Dorsey, S., Conover, K., & Burns, B.J. (2011). Parental Depression and Child Outcomes: The Mediating Effects of Abuse and Neglect. *Journal of Marriage and Family*, 73, 164–180.

Nicholson v. Scoppetta, NY Slip Op 07617, 3 NY3d 257 (2004).

Ondersma, S.J. (2002). Predictors of Neglect within Low-SES Families: The Importance of Substance Abuse. *American Journal of Orthopsychiatry*, 72 (3), 383–391.

Payne, M. (2014). *Modern Social Work Theory*, 4th edition. New York: Oxford University Press.

Perry, B.D. (1996). Neurodevelopmental Adaptations to Violence: How Children Survive the Intergenerational Vortex of Violence. *The Child Trauma Academy*. Retrieved from: www.childtrauma.org.

Perry, B.D. (2001a). Bonding and Attachment in Maltreated Children: Consequences of Emotional Neglect in Childhood. *The Child Trauma Academy*. Retrieved from: www.childtrauma.org.

Perry, B.D. (2001b). Violence and Childhood: How Persisting Fear Can Alter the Developing Child's Brain. *The Child Trauma Academy*. Retrieved from: www. childtrauma.org.

Perry, B.D. & Pollard, D. (1997). *Altered Brain Development Following Global Neglect in Early Childhood*. Society For Neuroscience: Proceedings from Annual Meeting, New Orleans.

Perry, B.D. & Szalavitz, M. (2006). *The Boy Who Was Raised as a Dog*. New York: Basic Books.

Read, J., Fosse, R., Moskowitz, A., & Perry, B.D. (2014). Traumagenic Neurodevelopmental Model of Psychosis Revisited. *Neuropsychiatry* 4 (1), 1–15.

Renner, L.M. & Slack, K.S. (2006). Intimate Partner Violence and Child Maltreatment: Understanding Intra- and Intergenerational Connections. *Child Abuse and Neglect*, 30 (6), 599–617.

Shepard, M. & Raschick, M. (1999). How Child Welfare Workers Assess and Intervene around Issues of Domestic Violence. *Child Maltreatment*, 4 (2), 148–156.

Sherman, B.F. & Holden, E.W. (2000). How Do I Assess Child and Youth Behavior? In H. Dubowitz & D. DePanfilis (Eds.), *Handbook for Child Protection Practice*, 273–277. Thousand Oaks, CA: Sage.

Shonkoff, J.P. & Phillips, D. (2000). *From Neurons to Neighborhoods: The Science of Early Childhood Development*. Washington, DC: National Academy Press.

Smith, M.G. & Fong, R. (2004). *The Children of Neglect: When No One Cares*. New York: Brunner-Routledge.

Thomlison, B. (1997). Risk and Protective Factors in Child Maltreatment. In M.W. Fraser (Ed.), *Risk and Resilience in Childhood: An Ecological Perspective*, 50–72. Washington, DC: NASW Press.

US DHHS (US Department of Health and Human Services). (2010). *Child Maltreatment 2010: Reports from the States to the National Child Abuse and Neglect Data System*. Washington, DC: US Government Printing Office.

US DHHS (US Department of Health and Human Services). (2013). *Child Maltreatment 2013: Reports from the States to the National Child Abuse and Neglect Data System*. Washington, DC: US Government Printing Office.

US DHHS (US Department of Health and Human Services). (2016). *Child Maltreatment 2016: Reports from the States to the National Child Abuse and Neglect Data System*. Washington, DC: US Government Printing Office.

US DHHS, Children's Bureau. (2011). Child Maltreatment 2010. *US Department of Health and Human Services, Administration for Children and Families, Administration on Children, Youth and Families*. Retrieved February 2012 from: http://www.acf.hhs.gov/programs/cb/pubs/cm10.

US Government Accountability Office. (2011). Child Maltreatment: Strengthening National Data on Child Fatalities Could Aid in Prevention. *GAO: US Government Accountability Office*. Retrieved February 2012 from: http://www.gao.gov/assets/330/320774.pdf.

WHO (World Health Organization). (2016). *Child Maltreatment*. Retrieved from: http://www.who.int/mediacentre/factsheets/fs150/en/.

Zipper, I.N. & Simeonsson, R.J. (1997). Promoting the Development of Young Children with Disabilities. In M.W. Fraser (Ed.), *Risk and Resilience in Childhood: An Ecological Perspective*, 244–264. Washington, DC: National Association of Social Workers Press.

Zuravin, S. (2001). Issues Pertinent to Defining Child Neglect. In T.D. Morton & B. Salovitz (Eds.), *The CPS Response to Child Neglect: An Administrator's Guide to Theory, Policy, Program Design, and Case Practice*, 1–22. Duluth, GA: National Resource Center on Child Maltreatment.

Zuravin, S. & DiBlasio, F. (1996). The Correlates of Child Physical Abuse and Neglect by Adolescent Mothers. *Journal of Family Violence*, 11 (2), 149–166.

6 Physical Abuse

Definition of Physical Abuse

The Center for Disease Control (CDC) defines child abuse as an act of commission.

> Acts of commission are deliberate and intentional; however, harm to a child might not be the intended consequence. Intention only applies to caregiver acts—not the consequences of those acts. The following types of maltreatment involve acts of commission: physical abuse, sexual abuse, and psychological abuse.
>
> (CDC, 2016, para. 2)

Physical abuse can include inflicting physical injury upon a child, including burning, hitting, punching, shaking, kicking, beating, throwing, stabbing, choking, or hitting with objects (CDC, 2016). There are always interactional variables involved in physical abuse. It is never just one thing that leads to the abuse. Environmental stressors; life stressors; and social, cultural, and economic factors are all variables to consider in physical abuse cases. This chapter focuses on physical abuse. Chapter 7 discusses psychological abuse, and Chapter 8 addresses sexual abuse.

Risk and Protective Factors

Risk factors are those factors that place a child at risk for maltreatment. When assessing physical abuse, social workers should be aware that it is never just one risk factor that places a child at risk. Multiple risk factors place additional stress on the parent or caregiver, which can create an environment where physical abuse can occur. Some of the risk factors social workers should look for include environmental and life stresses; unemployment; multiple moves; challenging relationships; poverty; little or no support; social, cultural, and economic difficulties; specific family characteristics;

family and interpersonal difficulties; parenting problems; inappropriate parental expectations; cultural influences; and a climate of violence in the home or in the community.

There are also protective factors that help mitigate the risk factors of physical abuse. Protective factors can include supportive relationships for both the child and parent or educational programs, which teach parents appropriate expectations for parenting and development (Goldman & Salus, 2003). Knowledge of parenting and child development provides parents with tools that support suitable expectations for communication, rules, and developmentally appropriate limits with children (Goldman & Salus, 2003; US DHHS, 2016). Parental resilience is another important factor. The ability to cope with life stresses helps a parent to respond to stress in a healthy manner instead of allowing it to impact parenting ability. Social connections and support are another protective factor. Connections can include friends, family, neighbors, community, and social service agencies. Social support provides parents with role models and children with opportunities for healthy interactions with adults (US DHHS, 2016). Providing the family with emotional and concrete supports, such as someone to talk to or services and resources, can lessen the stress on the parent. Additionally, nurturing relationships that promote attachment and provide relational-level protection assist in positive physical growth and brain development in babies and young children (US DHHS, 2016). The parent-child relationship is reciprocal. When children are able to self-regulate, communicate, and problem-solve, it has a positive impact on the parent (US DHHS, 2016).

Child Characteristics

Just as there are specific individual factors that promote protection, there are also specific characteristics that place children at higher risk for physical abuse. Younger children suffer more injuries from physical abuse than older children (Children's Bureau, 2016; Goldman & Salus, 2003). Physical abuse occurs similarly across all races; however, children with disabilities, specifically premature birth weight (Goldman & Salus, 2003) or physical, mental, or developmental disabilities tend to be at greater risk for victimization (ACF, 2012; Children's Bureau and NCANDS, 2009; Goldman & Salus, 2003). Additional characteristics that could contribute to physical abuse are children who have difficult temperaments or behavioral problems (Goldman & Salus, 2003).

Family and Parent Characteristics

There are also specific family and parent characteristics that place children at higher risk for physical abuse. Families living in poverty and large families tend to have higher rates of physical abuse (Klerman, 1993; Massat, 1995; NIS-4, 2006). Young parents (18–27 years old), low educational levels, and unemployment are factors that can contribute to physical abuse (Brown et al., 1998; Chaffin et al., 1996; NIS-4, 2006; Parrish et al., 2011; Putnam-Horstein & Needell, 2011). Families with deficits in parenting skills (Coohey, 1998; Koenig et al., 2000; Milner, 2000; Milner, 2003) or those where domestic violence is present are at greater risk for physically abusing (Children's Bureau and NCANDS, 2009; Zolotor et al., 2007). Additionally, female-headed families tend to have more incidents of physical abuse (Berger et al., 2009; Children's Bureau, 2016; Dufour et al., 2008; NIS-4, 2006; Sedlack et al., 2010). High stress levels from a variety of factors place children at higher risk for physical abuse, as does substance abuse by the parent (Dubowitz et al., 2011). Research has also found specific emotional and biological factors that place children at greater risk for physical abuse by a parent.

Emotional

Parents who physically abuse children tend to have difficulty controlling emotions, specifically anger and hostility. They have low frustration tolerance, low self-esteem, deficits in empathy, and rigidity (Mammen et al., 2003; Simons et al., 1991). Perpetrators may have a mental health diagnosis, such as depression or posttraumatic stress disorder (Pears & Capaldi, 2001). Antisocial personality disorder and maternal sociopathy have also been identified by researchers as factors associated with physical abuse (Brown et al., 1998: Capaldi, 1992; Capaldi & Stoolmiller, 1999).

Biological

Physiological traits also predispose parents to hyper-reactive responses or heightened physiological reactions to stressful stimuli, such as a crying child (Chen et al., 2010; McCormack et al., 2009).

Neighborhood Characteristics

A number of studies examined the association between community violence and child physical abuse. Lynch and Cicchetti (1998) found that physical abuse is related to the level of community violence. Other researchers have also linked neighborhood characteristics, like violence, to child maltreatment (Coulton et al., 1999; Freisthler et al., 2006).

Sibling Physical Abuse

Sibling physical abuse is another type of abuse that occurs within families but may not be assessed unless an obvious situation arises. This type of abuse is the most common form of abuse that occurs within families (Button & Gealt, 2010). Sibling fighting can be abuse and must be carefully assessed to verify if the fighting is within typical limits or has turned abusive. Sibling physical abuse is associated with substance abuse, delinquency, and aggression (Button & Gealt, 2010). When assessing for sibling physical abuse, social workers should look at the emotional and physical impact, severity, and intent of the abuse (Kiselica & Morrill-Richards, 2007). Sibling abuse has been related to other forms of family violence, such as intimate partner violence (Brody, 1998; Jenkins, 1992; Kiselica and Morrill-Richards, 2007; Noller, 2005), child maltreatment (Kiselica & Morrill-Richards, 2007), and controlling or hostile parent-child relationships (Brody, 1998). Sibling abuse can have long-term consequences. Victims can experience depression, insecurity, perceived incompetence, and low self-esteem (Hoffman & Edwards, 2004). Sibling abuse has also been tied to school violence (Duncan, 1999) and dating violence (Simonelli et al., 2002).

Assessment of Physical Abuse

An assessment for physical abuse has several components. Initially, a risk assessment is completed to determine whether the child can stay in the home with supervision or should be removed to ensure future safety. In addition to a social worker completing a multi-dimensional assessment, a physician should examine the child. More often than not, this examination is completed by an emergency room doctor, who is asked to determine whether the victim's injuries are due to physical abuse or not. Along with the examination, important information is also gathered in order for the physician to make the determination about the injury, such as the social context of the injury; information about the witnesses, like bias and motive; information about the circumstances; information about non-medical conditions that may look like abuse; labs, such as x-rays or blood work; details about the child, such as age and development; the child's medical history; and information about the parents or caregivers (Reece, 2011). Based on the outcome of the physical examination and the social work assessment, a determination in the case can be made. If physical abuse is the conclusion, the social worker will file the case with the court for a hearing.

Identifying Marks Caused by Physical Abuse

There are a variety of marks one might observe on a child's skin that could be indicators of physical abuse, including marks caused by instruments used

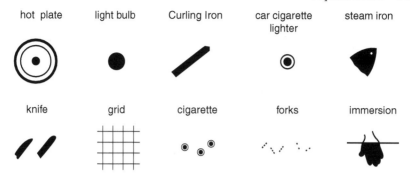

Figure 6.1 Marks from Burns

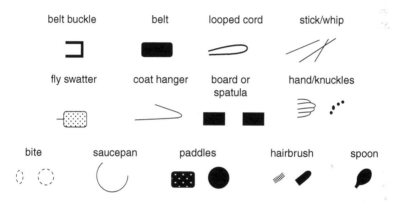

Figure 6.2 Marks from Instruments or Physical Contact

to inflict abuse or burns caused by implements or submersion in hot water. The following graphics depict the most common types of marks and the implements used to inflict the marks, such as burns (Figure 6.1), instruments or physical contact (Figure 6.2), bruises (Figure 6.3), immersion burns (Figure 6.4 and Figure 6.5), contact burns (Figure 6.6), and splash burns (Figure 6.7). Sometimes, social workers can view marks if they are located on arms and legs. However, sometimes marks are not readily visible because they are under clothing, on the back, or on the abdominal area. It is very important that a social worker does not physically examine a child under clothing or ask a child to remove clothing. This type of examination should only be done by a physician.

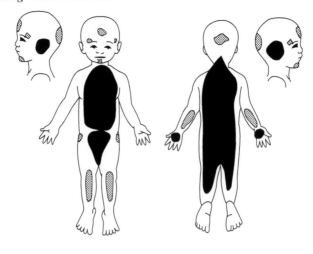

Low Suspicion [▒]

High Suspicion [■]

Figure 6.3 Bruises

Immersion Burn

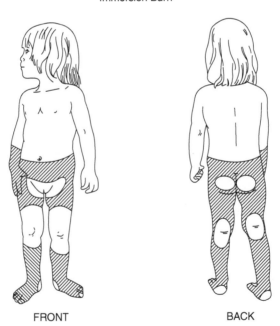

FRONT   BACK

Figure 6.4 Immersion Burn

Immersion Burn—How it Was Produced

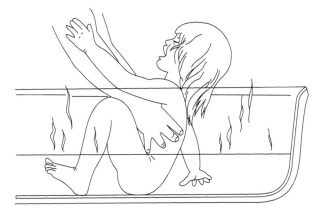

Figure 6.5 Immersion Burn

Contact Burn

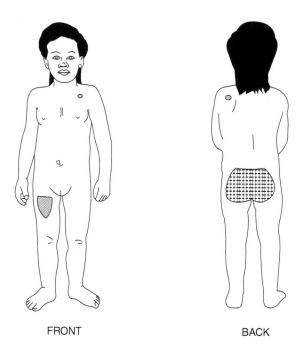

FRONT   BACK

Figure 6.6 Contact Burn

Splash Burn

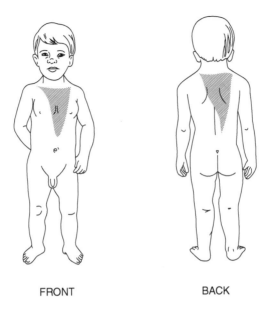

FRONT　　　　　　　　　BACK

Figure 6.7 Splash Burn

Cultural Practices

During an assessment, it is always important to consider the family's culture or cultural practices. Some cultural practices are generally not defined as physical abuse but may result in physical injury or harm. When assessing for physical abuse, it is important to consider cultural practices and be respectful of those practices. However, if the injury or harm to the child is significant, social workers should work with parents to discourage the harmful behavior and educate on alternatives that are not physically abusive (Dubowitz & Black, 2001). Below are some practices to be aware of when assessing physical abuse (Table 6.1).

Table 6.1 Cultural Practices

Type of Cultural Practice	Definition
Coining (cao gio)	a practice to treat illness by rubbing the body forcefully with a coin or other hard object that is dipped in hot oil
Moxibustion	Asian folkloric remedy that burns the skin
Caida de la Mollera (fallen fontanelle)	caused by holding a child upside down in order to treat vomiting and diarrhea—retinal hemorrhage can occur, which looks like shaken baby syndrome

Munchausen by Proxy Syndrome

A rare form of physical abuse is Munchausen by Proxy Syndrome (MPS). MPS occurs when a parent or caretaker (usually the mother) simulates or induces symptoms of physical illness in a child (i.e., suffocation, poisoning, etc.) (Eminson et al., 2000; Lasher & Sheridan, 2004). The parent takes the child in for medical treatment but denies the cause of the child's injuries. The child often experiences unnecessary medical treatment in order to find the cause of the illness (Eminson et al., 2000; Lasher & Sheridan, 2004). Victimization occurs over a long period of time. This type of physical abuse occurs because the parent or caregiver, in order to meet their own needs, uses the child to maintain relationships with medical personnel (Eminson et al., 2000; Lasher & Sheridan, 2004).

Misdiagnosis of Physical Abuse

During an assessment, it can be easy to misdiagnose physical abuse. Sometimes an accidental contact with an object, a fall, self-inflicted injuries, metabolic or infectious diseases, bleeding disorders, allergic skin reactions, and birthmarks can resemble marks associated with physical abuse. For example, cigarette burns look like impetigo, Mongolian spots look like bruising, ringworm looks like bite marks, and skin discoloration caused by markers, paint, etc., can look like bruising or marks from abuse. In addition to the above, there are also cultural practices to consider during the assessment of physical abuse.

Although an injury resulting from physical abuse is not accidental, the parent or caregiver may not have intended to hurt the child. The injury may have resulted from severe discipline, such as injurious spanking, or physical punishment that is inappropriate to the child's age. Injury may result from a single episode or repeated episodes, and it can range in severity from minor marks and bruising to death.

Consequences of Physical Abuse

Child victims of physical abuse can suffer medical and neurobiological problems; cognitive difficulties; behavioral and emotional issues; socio-emotional deficits (Runyon & Urquiza, 2011); mental health disorders, such as posttraumatic stress disorder (Saunders et al., 2004), depression (Kolko, 2002), or anxiety; and physical, behavioral, and emotional impairments, which can continue into adulthood (Goldman & Salus, 2003). Children who have experienced abuse may also model the abusive behavior with peers, lack empathy, and have poor impulse control (Perry, 2001).

Treatment of Physical Abuse

Treatment of physical abuse can vary and may depend on age. Initially, medical care to treat the child for injuries sustained from abuse may be required. Individual therapy, such as trauma-focused play therapy (Gil, 1996), therapeutic day care (Moore et al., 1998), or combined cognitive behavioral therapy (Donohue et al., 1998; Runyon & Urquiza, 2011) can be effective treatments for children who have been victims of physical abuse.

For parents, family therapy (Ralston & Swenson, 1996; Saunders & Meinig, 2000), parent-child interaction therapy (Eyberg, 1988; Runyon & Urquiza, 2011), and cognitive behavioral therapy (Runyon & Urquiza, 2011) are treatments proven to be effective. Additionally, in-home services (Fraser et al., 1996; Gershater-Molko et al., 2003), substance abuse programs, respite care programs, and parenting education can be effective interventions to prevent future physical abuse (Goldman & Salus, 2003). It is important to keep in mind that interventions should be sensitive to the family's culture. Social workers should be aware of values, beliefs, or customs that impact parenting and discipline in order to provide the best intervention possible (Goldman & Salus, 2003).

Case Examples and Questions

For each of the case examples, please answer the following questions:

1   Do you think physical abuse is occurring? And, if so, how would you classify the physical abuse you think is occurring (mild, moderate, severe, chronic)?
2   What risk and protective factors related to family, child, and parent characteristics seem to be relevant in this case?
3   What seems to be the parent's awareness of the important issues identified?
4   Is there prior involvement with the child welfare system?

   (A)   And, if so, how does it impact your assessment of the case?

5   What intervention(s) do you think should be provided to the family? Why?

Case One

During a violent fight between her parents, 8-year-old Melissa called 911. She told the operator that her father always hit her mommy when he came home drunk. In addition, Melissa said she was worried about her 5-year-old brother, Tommy. He tried to help their mom, and the father punched Tommy in the face while swinging at their mother. As a result, Tommy fell, hit his head on the coffee table, and had not moved since. The operator heard yelling in the background, and the mother screamed, "Get off the phone!" When the police and paramedics arrived, Tommy was unconscious, and the mother had numerous bruises on her face.

Case Two

John and his brother, Aaron, fight a lot. Sometimes Aaron ends up with bruises, and one time had to go to the hospital for a broken arm. John told his parents the broken arm was an accident. He had pinned Aaron to the ground and twisted his arm back like he had witnessed on the wrestling shows he watched. John also gets into trouble at school. He has been suspended for fighting with other children and has difficulty keeping his hands to himself. John and Aaron's parents have recently separated. The boys live with their mother because the father is in substance abuse treatment for 90 days. When the father lived in the home, he often disciplined the boys using harsh corporal punishment. Most times, the boys ended up with bruises or cuts afterwards.

References

ACF (Administration for Children and Families). (2012). *Child Maltreatment, 2011 Report.* Washington, DC: US Department of Health and Human Services.

Berger, L.M., Paxson, C., & Waldfogel, J. (2009). Mothers, Men, and Child Protective Services Involvement. *Child Maltreatment*, 14 (3), 263–276.

Brody, G.H. (1998). Sibling Relationship Quality: Its Causes and Consequences. *Annual Review of Psychology*, 49, 1–24.

Brown, J., Cohen, P., Johnson, J.G., & Salzinger, S. (1998). A Longitudinal Analysis of Risk Factors for Child Maltreatment: Findings of a 17-Year Prospective Study of Officially Recorded and Self-Reported Child Abuse and Neglect. *Child Abuse and Neglect*, 22 (11), 1065–1078.

Button, D.M. & Gealt, R. (2010). High Risk Behaviors Among Victims of Sibling Abuse. *Journal of Family Violence*, 25, 131–140.

Capaldi, D.M. (1992). Co-occurrence of Conduct Problems and Depressive Symptoms in Early Adolescent Boys: A 2-Year Follow-up at Grade 8. *Development and Psychopathology*, 4 (1), 125–144.

Capaldi, D.M. & Stoolmiller, M. (1999). Co-occurrence of Conduct Problems and Depressive Symptoms in Early Adolescent Boys: Prediction to Young-Adult Adjustment. *Development and Psychopathology*, 11 (1), 59–84.

CDC (Centers for Disease Control). (2016). Child Abuse and Neglect Definitions. *CDC: Centers for Disease Control and Prevention.* Retrieved from: http://www.cdc.gov/ViolencePrevention/childmaltreatment/definitions.html.

Chaffin, M., Kelleher, K., & Hollenberg, J. (1996). Onset of Physical Abuse and Neglect: Psychiatric, Substance Abuse, and Social Risk Factors from Prospective Community Data. *Child Abuse and Neglect*, 20 (3), 191–203.

Chen, H.Y., Hou, T.W., & Chuang, C.H. (2010). Applying Data Mining to Explore the Risk Factors of Parenting Stress. *Expert Systems with Applications*, 37 (1), 598–601.

Children's Bureau. (2016). *Child Welfare Outcomes 2010–2013: Report to Congress.* Washington, DC: Department of Health and Human Services, Administration for Children and Families. Retrieved from: https://www.acf.hhs.gov/cb/resource/cwo-10-13.

Children's Bureau and NCANDS. (2009). *Child Maltreatment 2009*. Washington, DC: US Department of Health and Human Services, Administration for Children and Families, Administration on Children, Youth and Families, Children's Bureau. Retrieved from: http://www.acf.hhs.gov/programs/cb/stats_research/index.htm#can.

Coohey C. (1998). Home Alone and Other Inadequately Supervised Children. *Child Welfare*, 77 (3), 291–310.

Coulton, C.J., Korbin, J.E., & Su, M. (1999). Neighborhoods and Child Maltreatment: A Multi-Level Study. *Child Abuse & Neglect*, 23 (11), 1019–1040.

Donohue, B., Miller, E., Van Hasselt, V.B., & Hersen, M. (1998). Ecological Treatment of Child Abuse. In V.B. Hasselt & M. Hersen (Eds.), *Sourcebook of Psychological Treatment Manuals for Children and Adolescents*, 203–278. Hillsdale, NJ: Lawrence Erlbaum.

Dubowitz, H. & Black, M.M. (2001). Child Neglect. In R.M. Reece & S. Ludwig (Eds.), *Child Abuse: Medical Diagnosis and Management*, 2nd edition, 339–362. Philadelphia, PA: Lea & Febiger.

Dubowitz, H., Kim, J., Black, M.M., Weisbart, C., Semiatin, J., & Magder, L.S. (2011). Identifying Children at High Risk for a Child Maltreatment Report. *Child Abuse and Neglect*, 35 (2), 96–104.

Dufour, S., Lavergne, C., Larrivee, M.-C., & Trocme, N. (2008). Who are These Parents Involved in Child Neglect: A Differential Analysis by Parent Gender and Family Structure. *Children and Youth Services Review*, 30 (2), 141–156.

Duncan, R.D. (1999). Peer and Sibling Aggression: An Investigation of Intra- and Extra- Familial Bullying. *Journal of Interpersonal Violence*, 14 (8), 871–886.

Eminson, M., Postlethwaite, R.J., & Eminson, D.M. (2000). *Munchausen by Proxy Abuse: A Practical Approach*. Woodburn, MA: Butterworth, Heinemann.

Eyberg, S.M. (1988). Parent-Child Interaction Therapy: Integration of Traditional and Behavioral Concerns. *Child and Family Behavior Therapy*, 10, 33–46.

Fraser, M.W., Walton, E., Lewis, R.E., Pecora, P., & Walton, W. (1996). An Experiment in Family Reunification: Correlates of Outcomes at One-Year Follow-Up. *Children and Youth Services Review*, 16, 335–361.

Freisthler, B., Merritt, D.H., & LaScala, E.A. (2006). Understanding the Ecology of Child Maltreatment: A Review of the Literature and Directions for Future Research. *Child Maltreatment*, 11 (3), 263–280.

Gershater-Molko, R.M., Lutzker, J.R., & Wesch, D. (2003). Project Safe Care: Improving Health, Safety, and Parenting Skills in Families Reported for, and At-Risk for Child Maltreatment. *Journal of Family Violence*, 18, 377–386.

Gil, E. (1996). *Treating Abused Adolescents*. New York: Guilford Press.

Goldman, J. & Salus, M.K. (2003). *A Coordinated Response to Child Abuse and Neglect: The Foundation for Practice*. Washington, DC: US Department of Health and Human Services, Administration for Children and Families, Administration on Children, Youth and Families, Children's Bureau, Office on Child Abuse and Neglect.

Hoffman, K.L. & Edwards, J.N. (2004). An Integrated Theoretical Model of Sibling Violence and Abuse. *Journal of Family Violence*, 19 (3), 185–200.

Jenkins, J. (1992). Sibling Relationships in Disharmonious Homes: Potential Difficulties and Protective Effects. In F. Boer & J. Dunn (Eds.), *Children's Siblings Relationships: Developmental and Clinical Issues*, 125–138. Hillside, NJ: Erlbaum.

Kiselica, M.S. & Morrill-Richards, M. (2007). Sibling Maltreatment: The Forgotten Abuse. *Journal of Counseling and Development*, 85, 148–161.

Klerman, L.V. (1993). The Relationship between Adolescent Parenthood and Inadequate Parenting. *Children and Youth Services Review*, 15 (4), 309–320.

Koenig, A.L., Cicchetti, D., & Rogosch, F.A. (2000). Child Compliance/Noncompliance and Maternal Contributors to Internalization in Maltreating and Nonmaltreating Dyads. *Child Development*, 71 (4), 1018–1032.

Kolko, D.J. (2002). Child Physical Abuse. In J.E.B. Myers, L. Berliner, J. Briere, C. T. Hendrix, C. Jenny, & T.A. Reid (Eds.), *The APSAC Handbook on Child Maltreatment*, 2nd edition, 21–54. Thousand Oaks, CA: Sage.

Lasher, L.J. & Sheridan, M.S. (2004). *Munchausen by Proxy*. New York: Haworth.

Lynch, M. & Cicchetti, D. (1998). An Ecological-Transactional Analysis of Children and Texts: The Longitudinal Interplay Among Child Maltreatment, Community Violence, and Children's Symptomatology. *Development and Psychology*, 10 (2), 235–257. doi:10.1017/S095457949800159X.

Mammen, O., Kolko, D., & Pilkonis, P. (2003). Parental Cognitions and Satisfaction: Relationship to Aggressive Parental Behavior in Child Physical Abuse. *Child Maltreatment*, 8, 288–301.

Massat, C.R. (1995). Is Older Better?: Adolescent Parenthood and Maltreatment. *Child Welfare*, 74 (2), 325–336.

McCormack, K., Newman, T.K., Higley, J.D., Maestripieri, D., & Sanchez, M.M. (2009). Serotonin Transporter Gene Variation, Infant Abuse, and Responsiveness to Stress in Rhesus Macaque Mothers and Infants. *Hormones and Behavior*, 55 (4), 538–547.

Milner, J.S. (2000). Social Information Processing and Child Physical Abuse: Theory and Research. In D.J. Hansen (Ed.), *Nebraska Symposium on Motivation*, vol. 45, 39–84. Lincoln, NE: University of Nebraska Press.

Milner, J.S. (2003). Social Information Processing in High-Risk and Physically Abusive Parents. *Child Abuse and Neglect*, 27, 7–20.

Moore, E., Armsden, G., & Gogerty, P.L. (1998). A Twelve Year Follow-Up Study of Maltreated and At-Risk Children Who Received Early Therapeutic Care. *Child Maltreatment*, 3, 3–16.

NIS-4. (2006). *The Fourth National Incidence Study of Child Abuse and Neglect*. Washington, DC: Administration for Children and Families, US Department of Health and Human Services. Retrieved from: http://www.nis4.org.

Noller, P. (2005). Sibling Relationships in Adolescence: Learning and Growing Together. *Personal Relationships*, 12, 1–22.

Parrish, J.W., Young, M.B., Perham-Hester, K.A., & Gessner, B.D. (2011). Identifying Risk Factors for Child Maltreatment in Alaska: A Population-Based Approach. *American Journal of Preventive Medicine*, 40 (6), 666–673.

Pears, K.C. & Capaldi, D.M. (2001). Intergenerational Transmission of Abuse: A Two-Generational Prospective Study of an At-Risk Sample. *Child Abuse and Neglect*, 25 (11), 1439–1461.

Perry, B.D. (2001). Violence and Childhood: How Persisting Fear Can Alter the Developing Child's Brain. *The Child Trauma Academy*. Retrieved from: www.childtrauma.org.

Putnam-Hornstein, E. & Needell, B. (2011). Predictors of Child Protective Service Contact Between Birth and Age Five: An Examination of California's 2002 Birth Cohort. *Children and Youth Services Review*, 33 (8), 1337–1344.

Ralston, M.E. & Swenson, C.C. (1996). *The Charleston Collaborative Project: Intervention Manual*. Charleston, SC: Author.

Reece, R.M. (2011). Medical Evaluation of Physical Abuse. In J.E.B. Myers (Ed.), *The APSAC Handbook on Child Maltreatment*, 3rd edition, 183–194. Thousand Oaks, CA: Sage.

Runyon, M.K. & Urquiza, A.J. (2011). Interventions for Parents Who Engage in Coercive Parenting Practices and Their Children. In J.E.B. Myers (Ed.), *The APSAC Handbook on Child Maltreatment*, 3rd edition, 195–212. Thousand Oaks, CA: Sage.

Saunders, B.E., Berliner, L., & Hanson, R.F. (Eds.). (2004). *Child Physical and Sexual Abuse: Guidelines for Treatment (Final report: January 15, 2004)*. Charleston, SC: National Crime Victims Research and Treatment Center.

Saunders, B.E. & Meinig, M.B. (2000). Immediate Issues Affecting Long-Term Family Resolution in Cases of Parent-Child Sexual Abuse. In R.M. Reece (Ed.), *Treatment of Child Abuse: Common Ground for Mental Health, Medical, and Legal Practitioners*, 36–53. Baltimore, MD: The Johns Hopkins University Press.

Sedlak, A.J., Mettenburg, J., Basena, M., Petta, I., McPherson, K., Greene, A., & Li, S. (2010). *Fourth National Study of Child Abuse and Neglect (NIS-4): Report to Congress Executive Summary*. Washington, DC: US Department of Health and Human Services.

Simonelli, C.J., Mullis, T., Elliot, A.N., & Pierce, T.W. (2002). Abuse by Siblings and Subsequent Experience of Violence within the Dating Relationship. *Journal of Interpersonal Violence*, 17 (2), 103–121.

Simons, R.L., Whitbeck, L.B., Conger, R.D., & Chyi-in, W. (1991). Intergenerational Transmission of Harsh Parenting. *Developmental Psychology*, 27, 159–171.

US DHHS (Department of Health and Human Services). (2016). *Building Community, Building Hope: 2016 Prevention Resource Guide*. Washington, DC: Administration for Children and Families.

Zolotor, A.J., Theodore, A.D., Coyne-Beasley, T., & Runyan, D.K. (2007). Intimate Partner Violence and Child Maltreatment: Overlapping Risk. *Brief Treatment and Crisis Intervention*, 7 (4), 305–321.

7 Psychological Abuse

Definition of Psychological Abuse

Sticks and stones will break my bones, but names will never hurt me. Have you ever had a broken bone or hurt yourself? Does it still hurt? Think of a time when someone may have called you a name or humiliated you. Does that still hurt? What would you say is worse, sticks and stones or names? Names can actually hurt more than sticks and stones. This is a good analogy for psychological abuse.

All states within the United States include psychological abuse somewhere in their legislation, often within legal definitions for child abuse or neglect. It is an "injury to the psychological capacity or emotional stability of the child as evidenced by an observable or substantial change in behavior, emotional response, or cognition as evidenced by anxiety, depression, withdrawal, or aggressive behavior" (Child Welfare Information Gateway, 2015, para. 8). Federal and state definitions are specific about what constitutes psychological abuse, and how a child will react in order to confirm abuse has occurred. Not all children react in the same way, although research points to some of the ways children may react. The CDC (2016) has a wider definition of psychological abuse. Psychological abuse occurs when a parent or caregiver's behavior harms a child's self-worth or emotional well-being (CDC, 2016). In essence, a parent or caregiver's behavior toward a child conveys to the child that they are worthless, flawed, unloved, unwanted, or in danger. Psychological abuse can be inflicted by using extreme or bizarre forms of punishment or threatening or terrorizing a child. It often goes hand-in-hand with other types of maltreatment. Psychological abuse is also known as emotional abuse, verbal abuse, or mental abuse.

Types and Severity of Psychological Abuse

There are many ways a parent can inflict psychological maltreatment on a child. Psychological abuse can be intentional or unintentional. It can be difficult to prove on its own. It often occurs with other types of maltreatment. The criteria between types of maltreatment overlap, and changes in a child's behavior may or may not be observable or substantial. It is also difficult to define when parental behavior becomes abusive. For example, when does grounding and sending a child to their room cross the line to become harmful isolating? Wolfe and McIsaac (2011) discuss a continuum of parental sensitivity and expression, which range from positive, healthy parenting behaviors to poor, dysfunctional behaviors that are abusive. Wolfe and McIsaac (2011) indicate that parents who fall in the middle of the continuum could benefit from parenting education, but they are not at a point that should be considered abusive. Intent and the severity of the psychological abuse are two considerations for assessing this type of maltreatment (Hamarman & Bernet, 2000). Both must be present in order for the behavior to be considered abusive. For example, where a parent deliberately degrades a child on a daily basis, there is intent to harm the child, and the maltreatment occurs frequently. Both intent and severity are present, which confirms that abuse is occurring. The table below lists different types of psychological maltreatments and how each may manifest (Table 7.1).

Table 7.1 Psychological Maltreatments

Type of Psychological Maltreatment	*Definition*
Denying emotional responsiveness	This occurs when a parent ignores a child or does not give appropriate emotional reactions to the child, including expressions of affection.
Exploiting or corrupting	Parental encouragement of inappropriate behaviors. This could be through modeling the behavior, permitting the behavior, or actively encouraging the behavior.
Isolating	Confining a child with little or no opportunity to socialize.
Mental health, medical, or educational neglect	Failing to provide for a child's mental health, medical, or educational needs.
Spurning	Verbal and non-verbal behaviors from the caregiver that are hostile and rejecting to the child. It can include belittling, degrading, shaming, ridiculing, and humiliating a child.
Terrorizing	Threatening violence or abandonment or placing a child in dangerous situations.

Source: (Myers, 2011)

Risk and Protective Factors

Denying emotional responsiveness and isolation are the most harmful types of psychological maltreatment for young children and adolescents, while verbal aggression or spurning are most detrimental for school-aged children (Brassard & Donovan, 2006; Goleman, 2006; Hart et al., 1998).

Parent or Family Factors

Family or parent characteristics that increase the risk for psychological abuse include caregivers who have difficulties or issues with interpersonal and social interactions, problem solving, or relationships. Psychological abuse can occur if the child was an unwanted pregnancy, if the parent has unrealistic expectations of the child, or if the parent was a young/teen parent. Parents who did not get their own childhood needs met, who have a need for emotional fulfillment from the child, or who have a need for emotional fulfillment in relationships also have a higher risk of psychologically abusing a child (Iwaniec, 2006). In some instances the child is an outlet for the parent's frustration or anger. Additionally, domestic violence (Moore & Pepler, 2006), parental substance abuse, or mental illness can be risk factors that place a child at a higher risk of psychological abuse.

Assessment of Psychological Abuse

Psychological abuse is the most difficult form of child maltreatment to identify. In part because the effects of psychological maltreatment, such as lags in development, learning problems, and speech disorders, are often evident in both children who have experienced abuse and those who have *not*. Additionally, the effects of psychological abuse may only become evident in later developmental stages of the child's life. Some indicators that psychological maltreatment has occurred can be identified through assessment of the child's behavior. Behaviors that indicate psychological maltreatment include mental health issues, such as anxiety, depression, suicide attempts, or low self-esteem (Binggeli et al., 2000; Binggeli & Hart, 2001; Brassard & Donovan, 2006; Caples & Barrera, 2006; Finzi-Dottan & Karu, 2006; Gibb et al., 2007; Iwaniec, 2006, Sachs-Ericsson et al., 2006); emotional problems, such as instability, substance abuse, or eating disorders (Binggeli et al., 2000; Binggeli & Hart, 2001; Brassard & Donovan, 2006; Garno et al., 2005; Iwaniec, 2006; McLewin & Muller, 2006); social issues; antisocial functioning; attachment problems; low empathy; withdrawing; aggression; delinquency (Binggeli et al., 2000; Brassard & Donovan, 2006; Crosson-Tower, 2009; Hughs & Graham-Bermann, 1998; Perry, 2001); learning problems (Binggeli et al., 2000; Brassard & Donovan, 2006; Hughs & Graham-Bermann, 1998); and physical symptoms or health problems (Binggeli et al., 2000; Bowlby, 1951; Brassard & Donovan, 2006; Crosson-Tower, 2009;

Spitz, 1956). Babies and young children may exhibit sleeping or eating problems, bed-wetting, mental health or emotional problems, apathy, crying and irritability, refusal to be calmed, and avoidance or little eye contact with adults, especially parents (Bowlby, 1951; Perry, 2001; Spitz, 1956).

Quantification of the parental behavior is also an important component of the assessment of psychological abuse. However, this can also be difficult. Unlike other types of maltreatment, psychological abuse is not always obvious or quantifiable. Evaluation of parental intent and the severity of the abuse are two ways to quantify psychological abuse. Assessing parental intent can be difficult to sort out. A parent may have good intention but still psychologically abuse their child. For instance, the parent may engage in a negative behavior with the child out of ignorance; however, abuse still occurred. Glaser (2002) indicates that, in order for psychological abuse to occur, a child's needs must not be recognized or respected by those who care for them. Severity is the second component of assessment of psychological abuse. Severity, or degree of harm, includes the frequency the maltreatment occurs, the duration of the maltreatment, and the intensity of the maltreatment. For example, a divorced parent repeatedly calls a child stupid and ugly because the child reminds the parent of the ex-partner. If this occurs over and over, and the parent has the intent to hurt the child, then both intent and harm are present. If intent and harm are both present, the maltreatment is considered severe (Hamarman & Bernet, 2000).

Measuring Psychological Abuse

One way to assess psychological abuse is to observe the mother-child relationship. Roth (1980) created the Mother-Child Relationship Evaluation. The evaluation outlines four types of relationship categories: accepting, overprotective, overindulgent, and rejecting. An accepting relationship is defined as having adequate affection, interest in a child's pleasure and activities, and an understanding of appropriate child development. The perception of the child is good in an accepting type of relationship (Roth, 1980). In an overprotective relationship, the mother experiences anxiety, prolongs infantile care, prevents development of independent behavior, and exerts excessive control (Roth, 1980). In an overindulgent relationship, the mother lacks parental control and is excessive in gratifying the child's wants or needs (Roth, 1980). In a rejecting relationship, the mother denies the child love, expresses hate in the form of neglect, is harsh, and can be brutal and strict (Roth, 1980).

There are other types of standardized measures available; however, none of these measures have high validity rates. Researchers reviewed 45 articles that examined 33 different measures of psychological abuse, and they concluded that while all of the measures had good reliability, none had been validated to ensure they measured what they said they measured (Tonmyr et al., 2011). However, in combination with other measures, like the

Childhood Trauma Questionnaire (Bernstein et al. 1994), a psychological abuse measure can be compared to enable more valid results. As well as using a standardized measure, social worker observation is an important component of the assessment process. Knowledge of child development and parent-child relationships is key to a factual and detailed description of the relationship, which can provide the evidence needed to ensure appropriate services for the child and family.

Consequences of Psychological Abuse

Psychological maltreatment is the strongest predictor of long-term impact on psychological functioning with long-term affects into adulthood. Some of these affects include antisocial behavior (Hart et al., 1998; Pearl, 1994); aggression (Loeber & Strouthamer-Loeber, 1986); psychological difficulties, such as anxiety, depression (Hart et al., 1998; Wright et al., 2009), withdrawal (Pearl 1994), low self-esteem (Briere & Runtz, 1990; Mullen et al., 1996), or self-abusive behavior (Erikson et al., 1989; Glassman et al., 2007); emotional problems or instability, such as personality disorders (Hart et al., 1998; Okado & Azar, 2011; van Harmelen et al., 2010); eating disorders (Hart et al., 1998; Rorty et al., 1994); learning problems (Doyle, 1997; Hart et al., 1998); and poor physical health (Gavin, 2011; Hart et al., 1998; O'Leary & Maiuro, 2001; Pearl, 1994; Spitz, 1956). On top of this large list of consequences, there is also an impact on the ability to attach.

Attachment is the formation of an emotional relationship with a caregiver. The relationship includes soothing, comfort, and pleasure (Perry, 2001). Children find security and safety in healthy attachments to parents and other caregivers. A healthy attachment is the basis for future healthy relationships with peers and intimate partners (Ainsworth, 1989; Ainsworth et al., 1978; Perry, 2001). Adequate and timely intervention is important in order to decrease the effects of psychological abuse and ensure that children have the ability to form a healthy attachment with their caregiver. Severe psychological abuse can impair a child for a lifetime. Children who have not formed a healthy attachment early on can lose the capacity to form meaningful relationships, struggle to develop normal relationships with others, and lose trust in others (Ainsworth, 1989; Ainsworth et al., 1978; Perry, 2001).

Treatment of Psychological Abuse

Case management and therapeutic services are highly recommended in psychological abuse cases. A case manager can oversee referrals and services for the child and parents as well as coordinate all providers and ensure compliance with treatment. Evidence-based therapeutic treatment is especially important. Parent-Child Interaction Therapy (PCIT) is an educational and coaching approach, which assists parents to respond to their children in a warm and nurturing manner (Hembree-Kigin & McNeil, 1995). School-based interventions can also be helpful, teach children pro-social behavior, and reinforce positive relationships with teachers. The *Incredible Years* teacher training series, for example, focuses on improving behavior management skills with teachers (Webster-Stratton, 2001). The *Dinosaur Social Skills and Problem-Solving* curriculum uses a group format to promote positive peer interactions, conflict resolution skills, and social competence (Webster-Stratton, 1991). Both programs are geared for pre-school-aged children. The *Primary Mental Health Project* is another program focused on internalized behaviors (Cowen, et al., 1996; Meller et al., 1994). This program is designed to develop a positive relationship between the provider and child while working on trust building and mutual respect. It has been found to increase self-confidence, enhance social problem-solving abilities, and reduce behavioral difficulties. Other pertinent services for families may include medical, legal, daycare, substance abuse treatment, and parental assistance services, such as a homemaking aid (Crosson-Tower, 2008).

Case Examples and Questions

For each of the case examples, please answer the following questions:

1   Is psychological abuse involved in this case? And, if so, how would you classify the psychological abuse you think is occurring (mild, moderate, severe, chronic)?
2   What risk and protective factors related to family, child, and parent characteristics, seem to be relevant in this case?
3   What seems to be the parent's awareness of the important issues identified?
4   Is there prior involvement with the child welfare system? And, if so, how does it impact your assessment of the case?
5   What intervention(s) do you think should be provided to the family? Why?

Case One

Tasha is a single parent raising Michael with no financial help from his dad. She gave birth to Michael when she was 17. Michael's parents tried to live together, but it just did not work out. The father moved out of the apartment and to another state several months ago. Michael is three years old. He is full of energy and constantly wants his mother's attention. Tasha is glad he is in daycare, because he wears her out. Tasha does not have a very good support system. She is estranged from her parents and has no siblings. She dropped out of school in her senior year and got a job after she had Michael. She relies on public housing and financial assistance to make ends meet. When Tasha plays with Michael she often feels self-conscious and immature. She feels Michael is at an age where he should be able to entertain himself, and she does not understand his need for constant attention and interaction with her when they are home together. When Tasha does play with Michael, she often teases him to the point that he cries. Tasha likes to pretend his elephant puppet is going to get Michael and often pushes this type of play. At daycare, Michael often complains of a stomachache at the end of the day when the children are starting to be picked up to go home.

Case Two

Lizzy is 12. Peers tease her at school because of her weight. She is tall and has always been larger than the other children. Lizzy's family is constantly telling her she is unhealthy and needs to lose weight. Even her pediatrician commented about her weight and the need for her parents to control her diet and food portions. Often, Lizzy's father, Robert, makes comments about her in front of others, such as family members, friends, and neighbors. He calls Lizzy "tub-o-lard" and "fatty". He says they are his pet nicknames for her. Although Lizzy's mom, Pat, does not call her names like her father does, she does use a different tone of voice when speaking to Lizzy and treats her differently compared to her siblings. Lizzy's mom weighs her every morning on the bathroom scale. If she has not lost any weight, Pat lectures Lizzy and tells her she will not get anywhere in life if she is obese. Pat says, "Obese people are just lazy people with no ambition. You don't want to be one of those people, do you?" Lizzy is withdrawn and very quiet. She has one friend at school and keeps to herself. The guidance counselor spoke to Lizzy and her parents about this. Her parents think she just needs to make more of an effort to be outgoing. After school, when her homework is completed, Lizzy's parents make her go outside. Pat tells Lizzy that she wants to see her actively playing with other kids in an effort to lose weight. Lizzy hides on the side of the house where her mother cannot see her and cries. She doesn't like to play with the neighborhood kids because they tease her and call her "Lizzy, Lizzy, big fat sissy".

References

Ainsworth, M.D.S. (1989). Attachments Beyond Infancy. *American Psychologist*, 44, 709–716.

Ainsworth, M.D.S., Blehar, M.C., Waters, E., & Wall, S. (1978). *Patterns of Attachment: A Psychological Study of the Strange Situation*. Hillside, NJ: Erlbaum.

Bernstein, D.P., Fink, L., Handelsman, L., Foote, J., Lovejoy, M., Wenzel, K., Sapareto, E., & Ruggiero, J. (1994). Initial Reliability and Validity of a New Retrospective Measure of Child Abuse and Neglect. *The American Journal of Psychiatry*, 151 (8), 1132–1136.

Binggeli, N.J. & Hart, S.N. (2001). *Psychological Maltreatment of Children*. Thousand Oaks, CA: Sage.

Binggeli, N.J., Hart, S.N., & Brassard, M.R. (2000). *Psychological Maltreatment: A Study Guide*. Thousand Oaks, CA: Sage.

Bowlby, J. (1951). Maternal Care and Mental Health. *Bulletin of the World Health Organization*, 31, 355–533.

Brassard, M.R. & Donovan, K.L. (2006). Defining Psychological Maltreatment. In M.M. Feerick, J.F. Knutson, P.K. Trickett, & S.M. Flanzer (Eds.), *Child Abuse and Neglect: Definitions, Classifications, and a Framework for Research*, 151–197. Baltimore, MD: Paul H. Brookes.

Briere, J. & Runtz, M. (1990). Differential Adult Symptomology Associated with Three Types of Child Abuse Histories. *Child Abuse and Neglect*, 14, 357–364.

Caples, H.S. & Barrera, M. (2006). Conflict, Support, and Coping as Mediators of the Relationship Between Degrading Parenting and Adolescent Adjustment. *Journal of Youth and Adolescence*, 35 (4), 603–615.

CDC (Centers for Disease Control). (2016). Child Abuse and Neglect Definitions. *CDC: Centers for Disease Control and Prevention*. Retrieved from: http://www.cdc.gov/ViolencePrevention/childmaltreatment/definitions.html.

Child Welfare Information Gateway. (2015). Definitions of child abuse and neglect. *Child Welfare Information Gateway*. Retrieved from: https://www.childwelfare.gov/topics/systemwide/laws-policies/statutes/define.

Cowen, E.L., Hightower, A.D., Pedro-Carroll, J.L., Work, W., Wyman, P.A., & Haffey, W.G. (1996). *School-Based Prevention for Children at Risk: The Primary Mental Health Project*. Washington, DC: American Psychological Association.

Crosson-Tower, C. (2008). *Understanding Child Abuse and Neglect*. Boston, MA: Allyn and Bacon.

Crosson-Tower, C. (2009). *Exploring Child Welfare: A Practice Perspective*. Boston, MA: Allyn and Bacon.

Doyle, C. (1997). Emotional Abuse of Children: Issues for Intervention. *Child Abuse Review*, 6, 330–342.

Erikson, M.F., Egeland, B., & Pianta, R. (1989). The Effects of Maltreatment on the Development of Young Children. In D. Cicchetti & V. Carlson (Eds.), *Child Maltreatment: Theory and Research on the Causes and Consequences of Child Abuse and Neglect*, 647–684. New York: Cambridge University Press.

Finzi-Dottan, R. & Karu, T. (2006). From Emotional Abuse in Childhood to Psychopathology in Adulthood: A Path Mediated by Immature Defense Mechanisms and Self-Esteem. *Journal of Nervous and Mental Disease*, 194 (8), 616–621.

Garno, J.L., Goldber, J.F., Ramirez, P.M., & Ritzler, B.A. (2005). Impact of Childhood Abuse on the Clinical Course of Bipolar Disorder. *British Journal of Psychiatry*, 186 (2), 121–125.

Gavin, H. (2011). Sticks and Stones May Break My Bones: The Effects of Emotional Abuse. *Journal of Aggression, Maltreatment, and Trauma*, 20, 503–529.

Gibb, B.E., Chelminski, I., & Zimmerman, M. (2007). Childhood Emotional, Physical, and Sexual Abuse and Diagnoses of Depressive and Anxiety Disorders in Adult Psychiatric Patients. *Depression and Anxiety*, 24, 256–263.

Glaser, D. (2002). Emotional Abuse and Neglect (Psychological Maltreatment): A Conceptual Framework. *Child Abuse and Neglect*, 26, 697–714.

Glassman, L.H., Weierich, M.R., Hooley, J.M., Deliberto, T.L., & Nock, M.K. (2007). Child Maltreatment, Non-Suicidal Self-Injury, and the Mediating Role of Self-Criticism. *Behavior, Research, and Therapy*, 45, 2483–2490.

Goleman, D. (2006). *Social Intelligence: The Revolutionary New Science of Human Relations*. New York: Bantam Books.

Hamarman, S. & Bernet, W. (2000). Evaluating and Reporting Emotional Abuse in Children: Parent-Based, Action-Based Focus Aids in Clinical Decision-Making. *Journal of the American Academy of Child and Adolescent Psychiatry*, 39 (7), 928–934.

Hart, S.N., Binggeli, N.J., & Brassard, M.R. (1998). Evidence for the Effects of Psychological Maltreatment. *Journal of Emotional Abuse*, 1 (1), 27–58.

Hembree-Kigin, T.L. & McNeil, C.B. (1995). *Parent-Child Interaction Therapy*. New York: Plenum Press.

Hughs, H.M. & Graham-Bermann, S.A. (1998). Children of Battered Women: Impact of Emotional Abuse on Adjustment and Development. *Journal of Emotional Abuse*, 1 (2), 23–50.

Iwaniec, D. (2006). *Emotionally Abused and Neglected Children*. Hoboken, NJ: John Wiley and Sons.

Loeber, R. & Strouthamer-Loeber, M. (1986). Family Factors as Correlates and Predictors of Juvenile Conduct Problems and Delinquency. In M. Tonry & N. Morris (Eds.), *Crime and Justice: An Annual Review of the Research*, vol. 7, 29–149. Chicago, IL: University of Chicago Press.

McLewin, L.A. & Muller, R.T. (2006). Attachment and Social Support in the Prediction of Psychopathology Among Young Adults With and Without a History of Physical Maltreatment. *Child Abuse and Neglect*, 30 (2), 171–191.

Meller, P.J., LaBoy, W., Rothwax, Y., Fritton, J., & Mangual, J. (1994). *Community School District Four: Primary Mental Health Project, 1990–1994*. New York: Community School District Four.

Moore, T.E. & Pepler, D.J. (2006). Wounding Words: Maternal Verbal Aggression and Children's Adjustment. *Journal of Family Violence*, 21 (1), 89–93.

Mullen, P.E., Martin, J.L., Anderson, J.C., Romans, S.E., & Herbison, G.P. (1996). The Long-Term Impact of Physical, Emotional, and Sexual Abuse of Children: A Community Study. *Child Abuse and Neglect*, 20, 7–21.

Myers, J.E.B. (Ed.). (2011). *The APSAC Handbook on Child Maltreatment*, 3rd edition. Thousand Oaks, CA: Sage.

Okado, Y. & Azar, S.T. (2011). The Impact of Extreme Emotional Distress in the Mother-Child Relationship on the Offspring's Future Risk of Maltreatment Perpetration. *Journal of Family Violence*, 26, 439–452.

O'Leary, K.D. & Maiuro, R.D. (Eds.). (2001). *Psychological Abuse in Violent Domestic Relations*. New York: Springer.

Pearl, P.S. (1994). Emotional Abuse. In J.A. Monteleone & A.E. Brodeur (Eds.), *Child Maltreatment: A Clinical Guide and Reference*, 259–283. St. Louis, MO: G.W. Medical Publishing.

Perry, B.D. (2001). Bonding and Attachment in Maltreated children: Consequences of Emotional Neglect in Childhood. *Childtrauma.org*. Retrieved from: https://childtrauma.org/wp-content/uploads/2014/01/Bonding-and-Attachment.pdf.

Rorty, M., Yager, J., & Rossotto, E. (1994). Childhood Sexual, Physical, and Psychological Abuse in Bulimia Nervosa. *American Journal of Psychiatry*, 151 (8), 1122–1126.

Roth R.M. (1980). *The Mother-Child Relationship Evaluation*. Los Angeles, CA: Western Psychological Services.

Sachs-Ericsson, N., Verona, E., Joiner, T., & Preacher, K.J. (2006). Parental Verbal Abuse and the Mediating Role of Self-Criticism in Adult Internalizing Disorders. *Journal of Affective Disorders*, 93 (1–3), 71–78.

Spitz, R. (1956). The Influence of the Mother-Child Relationship, and Its Disturbances. *Mental Health and Infant Development*, 1, 103–108.

Tonmyr, L., Draca, J., Crain, J., & MacMillan, H.L. (2011). Measurement of Emotional/Psychological Child Maltreatment: A Review. *Child Abuse and Neglect*, 35, 767–782.

van Harmelen, A.L., van Tol, M.-J., van der Wee, N.J.A., Veltman, D.J., Aleman, A., Spinhoven, P., van Buchem, M.A., Zitman, F.G., Pennix, B.W.J.H., & Elzinga, B.M. (2010). Reduced Medial Prefrontal Cortex Volume in Adults Reporting Childhood Emotional Maltreatment. *Biological Psychiatry*, 68, 832–838.

Webster-Stratton, C. (1991). *Dinosaur Social Skills and Problem-Solving Training Manual*. Seattle, WA: Incredible Years.

Webster-Stratton, C. (2001). *The Incredible Years: Parents, Teachers, and Children Manual*. Seattle, WA: Incredible Years.

Wolfe, D.A & McIsaac, C. (2011). Distinguishing Between Poor/Dysfunctional Parenting and Child Emotional Maltreatment. *Child Abuse and Neglect*, 35, 802–813.

Wright, M.O., Crawford, E., & Del Castillo, D. (2009). Childhood Emotional Maltreatment and Later Psychological Distress Among College Students: The Mediating Role of Maladaptive Schemas, *Child Abuse and Neglect*, 33, 59–68.

8   Sexual Abuse

Definition of Sexual Abuse

In 2005, 76% of reported sexual abuse perpetrators were friends or neighbors of the victims (Children's Bureau and NCANDS, 2009). Sexual abuse can occur within the family (intrafamilial) or outside of the family (extrafamilial). Sexual abuse is defined by the CDC (2016) as engaging children in sexual acts. More specifically, it is

> the employment, use, persuasion, inducement, enticement, or coercion of any child to engage in, or assist any other person to engage in, any sexually explicit conduct or simulation of such conduct for the purpose of producing a visual depiction of such conduct.
> (Child Abuse Prevention and Treatment Act of 2010, 2010)

Additionally, it can include, "the rape, and in cases of caretaker or interfamilial relationships, statutory rape, molestation, prostitution, or other form of sexual exploitation of children, or incest with children" (Child Abuse Prevention and Treatment Act of 2010, 2010).

Child sexual abuse generally refers to sexual behavior which includes a wide range of acts, such as oral, anal, or genital penile penetration; anal or genital digital or other penetration; genital contact with no intrusion; fondling of a child's breasts or buttocks; exposure to pornography; indecent exposure; inadequate or inappropriate supervision of a child's voluntary sexual activities; and/or use of a child in prostitution, pornography, internet crimes, or other sexually exploitative activities. Sexual abuse includes both touching offenses (fondling or sexual intercourse) and non-touching offenses (exposing a child to pornographic materials) and can involve varying degrees of violence and emotional trauma (Berliner, 2011; Crosson-Tower, 2008; Stein, 1998).

Although Faller (2002) indicates that the most commonly reported cases of sexual abuse involve incest, other researchers have found that an acquaintance or other person known to a child is the most common (Berliner, 2011; Finkelhor et al., 2009; Finkelhor et al., 2005; Saunders et al., 1999; Tjaden & Thoennes, 2000). Incest is sexual abuse occurring among family members (intrafamilial), including those in biological families, adoptive families, and step-families. Incest most often occurs within a father-daughter relationship; however, mother-son, father-son, and sibling-sibling incest also occurs (Berliner, 2011). Sexual abuse is also sometimes committed by other relatives or caretakers, such as aunts, uncles, grandparents, cousins, or the boyfriend or girlfriend of a parent (Finkelhor, 1984; Wiehe, 1997).

Risk and Protective Factors

Risk Factors

Finkelhor (2008) indicates that the type of trauma a child experiences is less important than the accumulation of trauma. The more trauma the child experiences, the higher the risk for negative effects in childhood and into adulthood (Dong et al., 2004). Berliner (2011) discusses three main factors that contribute to risk of persistent harm from sexual abuse: (1) pre-abuse risk factors, (2) nature of the abuse, and (3) the response when a child discloses sexual abuse. The first main factor, pre-abuse risk factors, includes prior trauma, mental health or emotional issues, and anxiety (Berliner, 2011). In addition, some family characteristics, such as parental mental or physical illness and domestic violence, add to the difficulty children experience later (Fitzgerald et al., 2008). The second risk factor, the nature of the abuse, can be described as the intensity and frequency of the sexual abuse. Some researchers have found that the perception of danger (Saunders et al., 1999) or violence during the abuse is associated with more negative outcomes for the child (Ruggiero et al., 2000). The third risk factor involves sexual abuse disclosure. When a child discloses sexual abuse, the initial response from the trusted adult can determine the level of trauma the child experiences. Negative responses from the trusted adult have been associated with higher levels of trauma (Bernard-Bonnin et al., 2008; Leifer et al., 1993; Mannarino & Cohen, 1997).

Child Characteristics

Child victims of sexual abuse are more likely to be female (Berliner, 2011; Fergusson & Mullen, 1999; Finkelhor, 1994; Gault-Sherman et al., 2009) and between the ages of 7 and 13 years old (Berliner & Elliott, 2002). However, a child can be sexually abused at any age. Lack of parental supervision and parental involvement is another risk factor found in families where sexual abuse is an issue (Elliott et al., 1995; Finkelhor, 1994). Children are also at greater risk of sexual abuse if they live with only one parent (Berliner & Elliott, 2002), have a cognitive or physical impairment (Berliner

& Elliott, 2002), have low self-esteem or lack self-confidence (Elliott et al., 1995), or they are overly compliant children (Gudjonsson et al., 2011).

Family or Parent Characteristics

The Children's Bureau and NCANDS (2009) found that 33% of parents/ relatives committed sexual abuse. Additional factors from the study indicated significant levels of dysfunction in the family, family violence and spouse abuse, conflicted and poor relationships, marital conflict, divorce, disorganized families that lacked cohesion and involvement with one another, deficient community involvement and support, problems with communication, lack of emotional closeness, and inflexibility. Mothers were often co-victims rather than co-perpetrators. Many times mothers were psychologically and physically abused as children (Finkelhor, 1994). Mothers were found to contribute to child victimization by withdrawing from the child or being unavailable. In addition, mothers tended to gravitate towards either men who were similar to their abusers or men who did not make sexual demands on them (Finkelhor, 1994).

The most predominant form of sexual abuse is contact between individuals where the perpetrator has a familial relationship with the victim (Finkelhor, 1994). Psychological trauma arises from incest due to the violation of the child's trust in the adult. Trauma from incest becomes worse the longer the abuse occurs. After disclosure, support from the mother or other significant adults is crucial.

Perpetrator Characteristics

Family members or individuals known to a child tend to sexually abuse more often than strangers (Berliner & Elliott, 2002). Males abuse more often than females (Finkelhor, 1984; Sedlak et al., 2010). Children living with both parents have the lowest risk of sexual abuse compared to children living with single parents (Sedlak et al., 2010). Often, the mother is absent due to illness, disability, or employment (Finkelhor, 1979; Finkelhor, 1984). A stepfather in the home or the absence of one or both biological parents is often found in families who sexually abuse (Friedrich, 1993; Goldman & Salus, 2003; Sedlak et al., 2010). Typically, the victim and the parents have a poor relationship, and often parental conflict or violence is present. Sexual abuse tends to occur more often in families with substance abuse issues (Goldman & Salus, 2003). The perpetrator often has a childhood history of physical, emotional, or sexual abuse (Crosson-Tower, 2008; Flora, 2001; Karson, 2001; Rich, 2006). Abusers engage in deviant sexual behavior, have difficulty forming healthy relationships, have low self-esteem, demonstrate poor social skills, and are unable to empathize (Crosson-Tower, 2008; Flora, 2001; Groth, 2002; Karson, 2001; Rich, 2006).

Other types of perpetrators include women and juveniles. It is suspected that there are more of these types of cases than known because they are underreported. Women typically engage in sexual abuse for several reasons according to Mathews et al. (1990). Some repeat the abuse they experienced themselves, some partner with a male perpetrator, some seek closeness with their victims, some have a need for power, and some see children as safe targets for displaced feelings. According to Ogilvie (2004), motivations to sexually abuse differ between males and females. Men tend to abuse for sexual satisfaction, while women abuse to meet emotional needs. For example, Mary Kay Letourneau was a 36-year-old teacher who molested her 13-year-old male student. They met when the child was in her second grade class. Letourneau spent 7.5 years in prison for the crime. It was one of the first publicized incidents of female sexual abuse.

Juvenile sexual offenders tend to offend for the first time at about 14 years of age. They have suffered sexual abuse and tend to assault children younger than themselves (Erooga & Masson, 2006). Many juvenile sexual offenders are reactive, meaning they will not necessarily abuse others if treatment is provided (Gil & Johnson, 1993)

Male juvenile perpetrators tend to prefer female victims, and they often have histories of victimization as well as family dysfunction, attachment difficulties, and mental health issues. Juvenile perpetrators also frequently offend as adults and have developed deviant sexual interests prior to the age of 18. Early intervention is essential to prevent future perpetration.

Grooming and Phases of Sexual Abuse

"Grooming" is a term used to describe how a perpetrator identifies and preys on a child in order to sexually abuse. Grooming typically takes place in an environment where the child feels safe, such as the home, school, church, or during activities the child might be engaging in, such as sports. During grooming, the perpetrator works to establish a relationship with the child and often looks for children who are vulnerable (Beauregard et al., 2007; Conte et al., 1989). Eventually, the perpetrator distances the child from others (Craven et al., 2006). Perpetrators focus their attention on children who do not have good relationships with their parents, appear lonely, are in need of attention, or have been victimized before (Craven et al., 2006).

Perpetrators follow a predictable, progressive pattern involving engagement, sexual interaction, secrecy, disclosure, and suppression (Craven et al, 2006; Lyon & Ahern, 2011). The progression of sexual abuse typically begins with sexual talk (Shannon, 2008) and leads to nonsexual touching, sexual touching, "accidently" seeing the child naked, or the child seeing the perpetrator naked (Craven et al., 2006; Kaufman et al., 1998). From this point, the perpetrator continues advancing with sexual behavior, eventually leading to intercourse. At times, bribes or threats are used during the process in order to make the child comply and keep the abuse a secret (Craven et al., 2006; Kaufman et al., 1998).

The US Gymnastics sexual abuse scandal is an example of sexual abuse perpetration outside of the family. For more than two decades, minor, female athletes were sexually abused by the team doctor. The abuse started in the late 1990s, and 368 individuals alleged they were sexually abused. In 2017, Dr. Larry Nassar pleaded guilty to federal child pornography charges and ten charges of first-degree sexual assault. In 2018, he was sentenced to an additional 40–175 years in prison after his initial 60-year federal prison sentence. As of 2019, Nassar is incarcerated at United States Penitentiary, Coleman. A nine-month investigation by *The Indianapolis Star* found that the abuses were widespread because "predatory coaches were allowed to move from gym to gym, undetected by a lax system of oversight, or dangerously passed on by USA Gymnastics-certified gyms" (Evans et al., 2016).

Sexual Exploitation

Sexual exploitation is often lumped into the same category as sexual abuse and, therefore, is important to discuss in this chapter as well. Definitions of sexual exploitation vary from state to state and country to country. Sexual exploitation can include all of the acts described above as well as engaging children in prostitution or in the production of child pornography. Exploitation generally involves money or financial gain (Mitchell et al., 2011). Perpetrators of child sexual exploitation can be parents, relatives, acquaintances of the child, or persons whose livelihoods involve exploiting children. The victims tend to be older children. They are often runaways, children who have been previously sexually abused, and children prostituting themselves independently.

Child Pornography

Child pornography is a federal crime, and all states have laws prohibiting it. It can be produced by anyone for personal use, trading, or sale on either a small or large scale. Copper (2009), found that 70% of all pornographic photographs of children were taken by close relatives or family friends. Pornography can also be used to instruct or entice new victims or blackmail those in the pictures. Production may be national, international, or local. The sale of child pornography is potentially very lucrative. Because of the availability of video equipment, digital cameras, and the internet, pornography is quite easy to produce and difficult to track. It is estimated that 20,000 new images are added to the internet each month (Copper, 2009). Keep in mind that pictures that are not pornographic or illegally obscene can nonetheless be very arousing to a pedophile. For example, an innocent picture of a naked child in the bathtub or even a clothed child in a pose can be used by a pedophile for arousal.

Child Prostitution

Child prostitution involves adults using minors to engage in sexual acts for money. Children with a history of maltreatment, those who have run away from home, or children who use alcohol or drugs are at higher risk for engaging in prostitution. Adolescent prostitution is more likely to occur in a sex ring, at the hand of a pimp, in a brothel, or with the child operating independently. Boys are more likely to be independent operators, while girls are more likely to be in involved in situations where others control the contact with clients. Oftentimes, child prostitutes are seen as criminals rather than victims (Lowe & Pearce, 2006).

Sex Trafficking

Similar to child prostitution, sex trafficking involves using children, usually for sexual acts for money. Child victims are coerced with kindness or promises or forced with intimidation, threats, or aggression (McClain & Garrity, 2011). Traffickers are well organized and target specific children. Child victims tend to come from isolated, dysfunctional, or poverty-stricken families (McClain & Garrity, 2011). Sex trafficking occurs in all countries, and victims are all races and ages.

Assessment of Sexual Abuse

There are several indications to be aware of when evaluating whether sexual abuse has occurred (Adams, 2000). The child victim may make a statement to a trusted peer or adult about the sexual contact. A caregiver may observe behaviors or notice physical signs on the victim that arouse a suspicion of sexual abuse. A health care provider may observe evidence of sexual abuse during an examination. A child victim may disclose sexual abuse during a therapy session. A child may have had contact with an individual who has been accused of sexual abuse. The child victim may be accused of perpetrating sexual abuse on another child.

Disclosure of Sexual Abuse

According to researchers, the failure to disclose sexual abuse is very common (London et al., 2005; Lyon, 2002; Lyon 2009; Paine & Hansen, 2002). Lyon and Ahern (2011) indicate that children often delay or fail to disclose sexual abuse if the perpetrator is a family member or someone known to the child. Inconsistencies during the disclosure process or the recanting of a disclosure is often due to the child's hesitancy to reveal the perpetrator rather than the child making a false accusation (Lyon & Ahern, 2011). Emotionality is also a factor in disclosing. Some children have feelings of embarrassment or shame, while others worry that they will be blamed for the sexual abuse (Anderson et al., 1993; Fleming, 1997). Some children do not want to upset others, or they feel a need to protect the perpetrator (Anderson et al., 1993).

Common Symptoms of Sexual Abuse

Symptoms of sexual abuse can be behavioral or physical or both. Physical symptoms may include injury evident on the genitals; sexually transmitted diseases; suspicious stains, blood, or semen on underwear, clothing, the body, or bedding; bladder or urinary tract infections; painful bowel movements or retention of feces; or early, unexplained pregnancy. The physical signs of sexual abuse are assessed during a medical examination. However, there may be no clear physical evidence depending on the time frame of the sexual abuse.

Behavioral symptoms vary from child to child and depend on the age. The child may verbally disclose the abuse, have sexual knowledge outside of the normal developmental age, engage in inappropriate sexual behavior, wear extra layers of clothing, not participate in normal physical activities, hide clothing, or exhibit emotional distress. The child may withdraw or become secretive, suffer from mood swings, cry for no reason, engage in self-harming behavior, or attempt suicide. Young children's sleeping or eating patterns may change. Older children may engage in sexually promiscuous behavior, set fires, or engage in animal abuse (Wickham & West, 2003). Some children may not display any behavioral symptoms at all (Faller, 2002; Wickham & West, 2003).

Assessment of sexual abuse differs significantly from other types of maltreatment. Knowledge of family roles in the abuse process is crucial in order to make a proper assessment. Assessment should include interviews with the child victim, perpetrator, family members, and other significant individuals such as doctor, teacher, or extended family. It is important to realize that the child victim may be stigmatized or rejected by the family, whose emotions (anger, denial, etc.) will be high.

Assessment data needed for the court process includes:

1   Physical evidence, such as medical findings and evidence collected by police.
2   Statements made to significant others. Most often sexual abuse comes to the attention of CPS through a significant other.
3   Sexual behavior by the victim, such as excessive masturbation, interaction with younger children/peers/other adults, seductive behavior, or sexual promiscuity.
4   Sexual knowledge beyond that expected for the child's developmental stage, such as knowledge of fellatio, intercourse, what happens to a penis when aroused, etc.

5   Nonsexual behavior indicators of stress, such as sleep disturbance; enuresis or incontinence; fear of sleeping in own room/bed; weight issues; change in dress; change in mood; or other regressive behaviors, including needing a pacifier or bottle, baby talk, clinginess, etc.

Medical Evaluation

Although protocol differs from state to state and country to country, a medical evaluation is an important part of the investigative process in a sexual abuse case. Medical evaluations are helpful to diagnose and treat the effects of sexual abuse and provide physical evidence of the sexual abuse for court proceedings (Finkel, 2011). An examination can also help ease concerns that the child victim or caregiver may have about the abuse and assist the child in the healing process (Finkel, 2011). Exams may be performed by specially trained physicians at a child advocacy center or by a pediatrician or emergency room doctor.

Three components are considered in medical evaluations for sexual abuse: the child and family history, a behavioral assessment, and a physical examination, which includes lab work to check for disease. Neither the physical examination nor the behavioral indicators stand on their own in court. Both need to support the history given by the child, which typically comes from a forensic interview by a specially trained interviewer.

Forensic Interview

When sexual abuse his been reported, disclosed, or substantiated, one component of the investigative process involves interviewing the child victim. Typically, interviews are conducted by a specially trained interviewer at a child advocacy center or in a similar environment. This type of setting is child-friendly and non-threatening. Forensic interviewers are trained to follow the National Institute of Child Health and Human Development (NICHD) interview protocol, which guides interviewers to use a narrative format (Sternberg et al., 2001) and to ask open-ended, non-leading questions rather than leading questions (Lamb et al., 2008).

Treatment of Sexual Abuse

Consequences of Sexual Abuse

Child victims of sexual abuse suffer a myriad of consequences. Most importantly, experiencing sexual abuse in childhood puts the victim at risk for many negative consequences in adulthood (Finkelhor et al., 1990). In his meta-analysis, Green (1993) found that emotional and mental health problems are common in children and include anxiety disorders, dissociation, hysteria, depression, low self-esteem, and disturbances in sexual behavior. Other researchers confirm emotional difficulties, most commonly depression and anxiety (Briere & Elliott, 2003; Caffo et al., 2005; Cohen et al., 2006; Lev-Wiesel, 2008; Maniglio, 2009; Putnam, 2003; Sapp & Vandeven, 2005, van der Kolk, 2005). Many researchers have found that children who have been sexually abused exhibit sexual behavior problems, such as developmentally inappropriate behavior (Friedrich, 1993), aggressive sexual behavior (Friedrich & Luecke, 1988), and sexually risky behavior (Fargo, 2009; Noll et al., 2009; van Roode et al., 2009).

Berliner (2011) confirmed Green's research and indicated that children who have been sexually abused feel intense fear and shame after the abuse. Avoidance of these feelings can lead to maladaptive behavior, such as numbing, self-harm, and risky behavior. Emotional issues, such as anger and depression, can develop and cause difficulties in interpersonal relationships (Chaffin et al., 1997). Trust in others can be lost, and assumptions about the child's self can become negative (Berliner, 2011; Daigneault et al., 2006; Feiring et al., 2007; Feiring et al., 2009; Mannarino & Cohen, 1997). In addition, eating disorders have been found at higher rates in children with a sexual abuse history than those children without (Wonderlich et al., 2000). Eating disorders can continue into adulthood and result in a variety of dysfunctional eating behaviors (Lock, 2009; Van Gerko et al., 2005).

As adults, victims continue to experience emotional and mental health issues (Briere & Elliott, 2003), suicidal behavior (Briere & Elliott, 2003; Dube et al., 2005; Fergusson et al., 2008; Greenfield, 2010; Horner, 2010), substance abuse (Berliner & Elliott, 2002; Duncan, et al., 2008; Maniglio, 2009; Shin et al., 2010; Moran et al., 2004), personality disorders (Goodyear-Brown et al., 2012), sexual problems (Briere & Elliott, 2003), revictimization, and sexual offending. In 2001, Paolucci, Genuis, and Violato completed a meta-analysis focused on specific outcomes from sexual abuse. They found that victims were at risk for posttraumatic stress disorder, depression, suicide, sexual promiscuity, poor academic performance, and involvement in a victim-perpetrator cycle of abuse (Paolucci et al., 2001). Greenfield (2010) also found overall poor physical health in adults who experienced childhood sexual abuse.

Most children recover from the consequences of sexual abuse; however, a small group of children do not. For instance, those victims involved in long court trials tend to have worsening symptoms (McCoy & Keen, 2014). Posttraumatic stress (PTS), the re-experiencing of the event, is reported at high levels in children who have been sexually abused (Finkelhor, 2008; McLeer et al., 1998). Children who have been sexually abused have higher rates of PTS or posttraumatic stress disorder (PTSD) than children who experienced other types of abuse (Berliner & Elliott, 2002; Deblinger et al., 1989; Dubner & Motta, 1999; Kilpatrick & Saunders, 1999; Putnam, 2003; Ruggiero et al., 2000). A big factor in recovery is family support and removal from the perpetrator.

Treatment for Child Victims

The degree of trauma the child experiences depends on the type of abuse, the identity of perpetrator, the duration of abuse, the extent of abuse, the age at which the child was abused, the first reactions of significant others at disclosure of the abuse (Feiring & Taska, 2005), the point at which the abuse was disclosed, and the personality of the victim. All of these factors should be considered before deciding on the type of treatment for a victim. Typical treatment for sexual abuse includes medical intervention (if needed), individual therapy, and group therapy. Research has found that some children, especially teens, do not require therapy. Finkelhor and Berliner (1995) found that up to 40% of children in one study had no symptoms related to sexual abuse. Kinnally et al. (2009) indicated that psychological resiliency comes from family support, a positive support network, and protective factors.

Specific treatment interventions for child victims can include play therapy, family treatment, cognitive behavioral therapy (CBT), or trauma-focused therapy. Play therapy helps the child reduce emotional distress through symbolic play (Webb, 1999). Family treatment is usually a combination of individual and family sessions. It focuses on strengthening the child-caregiver relationship and building family resilience (Sheinberg & Fraenkel, 2001). CBT incorporates education, skill development, safety skills training, and gradual exposure to abuse memories (Cohen et al., 2006). Lastly, trauma-focused therapy can consist of several types of therapeutic techniques. A popular technique is trauma-focused cognitive behavioral therapy (TFCBT), which includes both individual and family sessions and, like CBT, uses education, skills training, relaxation techniques, affective expression and modulation, coping, trauma narrative processing, in vivo mastery of trauma reminders, and enhancement of safety skills (Cohen et al., 2006).

Treatment for the Non-offending Parent/Caregiver

In addition to treatment for the child victim, the non-offending parent or caregiver may also be referred for treatment or other supportive services. Some interventions for the caregiver include identifying ways they can support and assist the child victim to manage difficult feelings or emotions (Deblinger & Heflin, 1996). Other interventions may provide support for non-offending mothers who may have been sexual abuse victims (Deblinger et al., 1994) or domestic violence victims (Deblinger et al., 1993).

Treatment for the Sexual Abuse Perpetrator

Adult Perpetrator

Treatment for adult sexual abuse perpetrators typically includes CBT within a relapse prevention model (Marshall, 1999; McGarth et al., 2003).

Conducted in a group format, CBT is used to analyze and challenge distorted thoughts in order to promote emotional and behavioral change (Kirsch et al., 2011). Treatment for perpetrators focuses on deviant sexual arousal, distorted cognitions, social skills, empathy, impulse control, emotional regulation, interpersonal relationships, substance abuse, and attitudes (Becker & Murphy, 1998). The goal of treatment is to reduce sexual abuse recidivism (Rice & Harris, 2003).

Juvenile Perpetrator

Like adult perpetrator treatment, juvenile treatment also uses CBT within a relapse prevention model as well as psychoeducation (McGarth et al., 2003). CBT with this population entails cognitive restructuring, victim awareness, empathy, anger management, social skills training, and sex education (McGarth et al., 2003). Multisystemic treatment (MST) is also used with juveniles. MST is a social ecological approach used for behavioral problems (Curtis et al., 2004). It is delivered in the home or community and utilizes strengths within the juvenile's systems to change behavior (Henggeler et al., 1998). Research has shown that any type of treatment for juvenile sexual perpetrators is effective in preventing recidivism (Kirsch et al., 2011).

Case Examples and Questions

For each of the case examples, please answer the following questions:

1   Which type(s) of sexual abuse may be involved in this case?
2   What risk and protective factors related to family, child, and parent characteristics seem to be relevant in this case?
3   What seems to be the parent's awareness of the important issues identified?
4   Is there prior involvement with the child welfare system?

   (A)   And, if so, how does it impact your assessment of the case?

5   Do you think sexual abuse is occurring?

   (A)   And, if so, how would you classify the abuse you think is occurring (mild, moderate, severe, chronic)?

6   What intervention(s) do you think should be provided to the family? Why?

Case One

Joanne took her 5-year-old daughter, Kendra, to the doctor after Kendra repeatedly complained about painful urination. During the examination Kendra cried when the doctor said she had to take off her clothes. Kendra told her mom that she felt better and didn't need a doctor. The examination revealed red, irritated, and swollen genitalia. She was also diagnosed with a yeast infection. The doctor asked Joanne if there had been any changes in Kendra's hygiene routine. Joanne stated that either her or her boyfriend bathed Kendra nightly. When asked about any changes in Kendra's behavior, Joanne related that on nights when she works she would come home and find Kendra sleeping in her snowsuit. Joanne's boyfriend is not Kendra's father, he does not live in the house, and they have only been dating for three months.

Case Two

Tom and Maggie Martin were called to meet with the school principal after their 7-year-old son, Zach, was caught masturbating in the school bathroom. Zach's teacher, Mr. Beck, reported that Zach asked several times during the day to go to the bathroom and was holding his crotch. After the fifth request, Zach was gone longer than normal, so Mr. Beck went to check on him. Mr. Beck observed Zach standing in front of the mirror with his pants down and masturbating. When the principal told Zach that kind of behavior is inappropriate, Zach replied, "Billy said it was normal and part of becoming a man." Billy is Zack's cousin who is in the tenth grade. Tom asked when Billy told him that, and Zach said it was during a family camping trip. Billy and Zack were given a boys' tent to set up and sleep in last weekend. Zach stated that the first night Billy showed Zach his erection and said that's how you become a man. The second night Billy showed Zach his erection and showed him how to play with it. Billy then asked Zach if he wanted to be a man. When Zach said yes, Billy told him to take his pants off. Once Zach started masturbating, Billy told him he wasn't doing it right and would help him. Billy then grabbed Zach's penis and instructed him how to masturbate.

References

Adams, J.A. (2000). How Do I Determine If a Child Has Been Sexually Abused? In H. Dubowitz & D. DePanfilis (Eds.), *Handbook for Child Protection Practice*, 175–179. Thousand Oaks, CA: Sage.

Anderson, J., Martin, J, Mullen, P., Romans, S., & Herbison, P. (1993). Prevalence of Childhood Sexual Abuse Experiences in a Community Sample of Women. *Journal of the American Academy of Child and Adolescent Psychiatry*, 32, 911–919.

Beauregard, E., Rossmo, D.K., & Proulx, J. (2007). A Descriptive Model of the Hunting Process of Serial Sex Offenders: A Rational Choice Perspective. *Journal of Family Violence*, 22, 449–463.

Becker, J.V. & Murphy, W.D. (1998). What We Know and Do Not Know about Assessing and Treating Sexual Offenders. *Psychology, Public Policy and Law*, 4, 116–137.

Berliner, L. (2011). Child Sexual Abuse. In J.E.B. Myers (Ed.), *The ASPC Handbook on Child Maltreatment*, 3rd edition, 215–232. Thousand Oaks, CA: Sage.

Berliner, L. & Elliott, D.M. (2002). Sexual Abuse of Children. In J.E.B. Myers, L. Berliner, J. Briere, C.T. Hendrix, C. Jenny, & T.A. Reid (Eds.), *The APSAC Handbook on Child Maltreatment*, 2nd edition, 55–78. Thousand Oaks, CA: Sage.

Bernard-Bonnin, A.C., Herbert, M., Daignault, I.V., & Allard-Dansereau, C. (2008). Disclosure of Sexual Abuse and Personal and Familial Factors as Predictors of Post-Traumatic Stress Disorder Symptoms in School-Aged Girls. *Pediatrics and Child Health*, 13, 479–486.

Briere, J. & Elliott, D.M. (2003). Prevalence and Psychological Sequelae of Self-Reported Childhood Physical and Sexual Abuse in a General Population Sample of Men and Women. *Child Abuse and Neglect*, 27, 1205–1222.

Caffo, E., Forresi, B., & Lievers, L.S. (2005). Impact, Psychological Sequelae and Management of Trauma Affecting Children and Adolescents. *Current Opinion in Psychiatry*, 18 (4), 422–428.

CDC (CDC). (2016). Child Sexual Abuse. *CDC: Centers for Disease Control and Prevention*. Retrieved from: http://www.cdc.gov/ViolencePrevention/childma ltreatment/definitions.html.

Chaffin, M., Wherry, J.N., & Dykman, R. (1997). School Age Children's Coping with Sexual Abuse: Abuse Stresses and Symptoms Associated with Four Coping Strategies. *Child Abuse and Neglect*, 21, 227–240.

Child Abuse Prevention and Treatment Act of 2010. (2010). 42 U.S.C. § 5106g.

Children's Bureau and NCANDS. (2009). *Child Maltreatment 2009*. Washington, DC: US Department of Health and Human Services, Administration for Children and Families, Administration on Children, Youth and Families, Children's Bureau. Retrieved from: http://www.acf.hhs.gov/programs/cb/stats_research/index.htm#can.

Cohen, J.A., Mannarino, A.P., & Deblinger, E. (2006). *Treating Trauma and Traumatic Grief in Children and Adolescents*. New York: Guilford Press.

Conte, J., Wolf, S., & Smith, T. (1989). What Sexual Offenders Tell Us About Prevention Strategies. *Child Abuse and Neglect*, 13, 293–301.

Copper, S.W. (2009). The Sexual Exploitation of Children and Youth: Redefining Victimization. In S. Olfman (Ed.), *The Sexualization of Childhood*, 105–120. Westport, CT: Praeger.

Craven, S., Brown, S., & Gilchrist, E. (2006). Sexual Grooming of Children: Review of Literature and Theoretical Considerations. *Journal of Sexual Aggression*, 12 (3), 287–299.

Crosson-Tower, C. (2008). *Understanding Child Abuse and Neglect*. Boston, MA: Allyn and Bacon.

Curtis, N.M, Ronan, K.R., & Borduin, C.M. (2004). Multisystemic Treatment: A Meta-Analysis of Outcome Studies. *Journal of Family Psychology*, 18, 411–419.

Daigneault, I., Tourigny, M., & Herbert, M. (2006). Self-Attributions of Blame in Sexually Abused Adolescents: A Meditational Model. *Journal of Traumatic Stress*, 19, 153–157.

Deblinger, E., Hathaway, C.R., Lippmann, J., & Steer, R. (1993). Psychosocial Characteristics and Correlates of Symptom Distress in Non-Offending Mothers of Sexually Abused Children. *Journal of Interpersonal Violence*, 8, 155–168.

Deblinger, E. & Heflin, A.H. (1996). *Treating Sexually Abused Children and Their Nonoffending Parents*. Thousand Oaks, CA: Sage.

Deblinger, E., McLeer, S.V., Atkins, M.S., Ralphe, D., & Foa, E. (1989). Post-traumatic Stress in Sexually Abused, Physically Abused, and Nonabused Children. *Child Abuse and Neglect*, 13, 403–408.

Deblinger, E., Stauffer, L., & Landsberg, C. (1994). The Impact of a History of Child Sexual Abuse on Maternal Response to Allegations of Sexual Abuse Concerning Her Child. *Journal of Child Sexual Abuse*, 3, 67–75.

Dong, M., Anda, R.F., Felitti, V.J., Dube, S.R., Williamson, D.F., Thompson, T.J., Loo, C.M., & Giles, W.H. (2004). The Interrelatedness of Multiple Forms of Childhood Abuse, Neglect, and Household Dysfunction. *Child Abuse and Neglect*, 28, 771–784.

Dube, S.R., Anda, R.F., Whitfield, C.L., Brown, D.W., Felitti, V.J., Dong, M., & Giles, W.H. (2005). Long-Term Consequences of Childhood Sexual Abuse by Gender of Victim. *American Journal of Preventive Medicine*, 28 (5), 430–438.

Dubner, A.E. & Motta, R.W. (1999). Sexually and Physically Abused Foster Care Children and Posttraumatic Stress Disorder. *Journal of Consulting and Clinical Psychology*, 67, 367–373.

Duncan, A.E., Sartor, C.E., Scherrer, J.F., Grant, J.D., Heath, A.C., Nelson, E.C., Jacob, T., & Keenan Bocholz, K. (2008). The Association Between Cannabis Abuse and Dependence and Childhood Physical and Sexual Abuse: Evidence from an Offspring of Twins Design. *Addiction*, 103, 990–997.

Elliott, D., Browne, K., & Kilcoyne, J. (1995). Child Sexual Abuse Prevention: What Offenders Tell Us. *Child Abuse and Neglect*, 19, 579–594.

Erooga, M. & Masson, H. (Eds.). (2006). *Children and Young People Who Sexually Abuse*. London: Routledge.

Evans, T., Alesia, M., & Kwiatkowski, M. (2016). A 20-Year Toll: 368 Gymnasts Allege Sexual Exploitation. *The Indianapolis Star*. Retrieved May 21, 2020 from: https://eu.indystar.com/story/news/2016/12/15/20-year-toll-368-gymnasts-allege-sexual-exploitation/95198724.

Faller, K.C. (2002). *Understanding Child Sexual Maltreatment*. Newbury Park, CA: Sage.

Fargo, J.D. (2009). Pathways to Adult Sexual Revictimization: Direct and Indirect Behavioral Risk Factors Across the Lifespan. *Journal of Interpersonal Violence*, 24, 1771–1791.

Feiring, C., Miller-Johnson, S., & Cleland, C.M. (2007). Potential Pathways from Stigmatization and Internalizing Symptoms to Delinquency in Sexually Abused Youth. *Child Maltreatment*, 12, 220–232.

Feiring, C., Simon, V.A., & Cleland, C.M. (2009). Childhood Sexual Abuse, Stigmatization, Internalizing Symptoms, and the Development of Sexual Difficulties and Dating Aggression. *Journal of Consulting and Clinical Psychology*, 77, 127–137.

Feiring, C. & Taska, L.S. (2005). The Persistence of Shame Following Sexual Abuse: A Longitudinal Look at Risk and Recovery. *Child Maltreatment*, 10, 337–349.

Fergusson, D.M., Boden, J.M., & Horwood, L. (2008). Exposure to Childhood Sexual and Physical Abuse and Adjustment in Early Adulthood. *Child Abuse and Neglect*, 32, 607–619.

Fergusson, D.M. & Mullen, P.E. (1999). *Childhood Sexual Abuse: An Evidence Based Perspective*. Thousand Oaks, CA: Sage.

Finkel, M.A. (2011). Medical Issues in Child Sexual Abuse. In J.E.B. Myers (Ed.), *The APSAC Handbook of Child Maltreatment*, 3rd edition, 215–232. Thousand Oaks, CA: Sage.

Finkelhor, D. (1979). *Sexually Victimized Children*. New York: Freepress.

Finkelhor, D. (1984). *Child Sexual Abuse*. New York: Freepress.

Finkelhor, D. (1994). Current Information on the Scope and Nature of Child Sexual Abuse. *The Future of Children*, 4 (2), 31–53.

Finkelhor, D. (2008). *Childhood Victimization: Violence, Crime, and Abuse in the Lives of Young People.* New York: Oxford University Press.

Finkelhor, D. & Berliner, L. (1995). Research on the Treatment of Sexually Abused Children. *Journal of the American Academy of Child and Adolescent Psychiatry*, 34, 1408–1423.

Finkelhor, D., Hotaling, G., Lewis, I.A., & Smith, C. (1990). Sexual Abuse in a National Survey of Adult Men and Women: Prevalence, Characteristics, and Risk Factors. *Child Abuse and Neglect*, 14 (1), 19–28. doi:10.1016/0145-2134(90) 90077-7.

Finkelhor, D., Ormrod, R., & Turner, H.A. (2009). Lifetime Assessment of Poly-Victimization in a National Sample of Children and Youth. *Child Abuse and Neglect*, 33, 403–411.

Finkelhor, D., Ormrod, R., Turner, H., & Hamby, S.L. (2005). The Victimization of Children and Youth: A Comprehensive, National Survey. *Child Maltreatment*, 10, 5–25.

Fitzgerald, M.M., Schneider, R.A., Salstrom, S., Zinzow, H.M., Jackson, J., & Fossel, R.V. (2008). Child Sexual Abuse, Early Family Risk, and Childhood Parentification: Pathways to Current Psychosocial Adjustment. *Journal of Family Psychology*, 22, 320–324.

Fleming, J.M. (1997). Prevalence of Childhood Sexual Abuse in a Community Sample of Australian Women. *Medical Journal of Australia*, 166, 65–68.

Flora, R. (2001). *How to Work with Sexual Offenders.* New York: Haworth.

Friedrich, W.N. (1993). Sexual Victimization and Sexual Behavior in Children: A Review of Recent Literature. *Child Abuse and Neglect*, 17, 59–66.

Friedrich, W.N. & Luecke, W.J. (1988). Young School-Age Sexually Aggressive Children. *Professional Psychology: Research and Practice*, 19, 155–164.

Gault-Sherman, M., Silver, E., & Sigfusdottir, I.D. (2009). Gender and the Associated Impairments of Childhood Sexual Abuse: A National Study of Icelandic Youth. *Social Science and Medicine*, 69, 1515–1522.

Gil, E. & Johnson, T.C. (1993). *Sexualized Children.* Rockville, MD: Launch Press.

Goldman, J. & Salus, M.K. (2003). *A Coordinated Response to Child Abuse and Neglect: The Foundation for Practice.* Washington, DC: US Department of Health and Human Services, Administration for Children and Families, Administration on Children, Youth and Families, Children's Bureau, Office on Child Abuse and Neglect.

Goodyear-Brown, P., Faith, A., & Myers, L. (2012). Child Sexual Abuse: The Scope of the Problem. In P. Goodyear-Brown (Ed.), *Handbook of Child Sexual Abuse: Identification, Assessment, and Treatment*, 3–28. Hoboken, NJ: John Wiley and Sons.

Green, A.H. (1993). Child Sexual Abuse: Immediate and Long-Term Effects and Intervention. *Journal of the American Academy of Child and Adolescent Psychiatry*, 32 (5), 890–902.

Greenfield, E.A. (2010). Child Abuse as a Life-Course Determinant of Adult Health. *Maturitas*, 66, 51–55.

Groth, A.N. (2002). *Men Who Rape.* New York: Perseus Press.

Gudjonsson, G.H., Sigurdsson, J.F., & Tryggvadottir, H.B. (2011). The Relationship of Compliance With a Background of Childhood Neglect and Physical and Sexual Abuse. *The Journal of Forensic Psychiatry & Psychology*, 22 (1), 87–98.

Henggeler, S.W., Schoenwald, S.K., Borduin, C.M., Rowland, M.D., & Cunningham, P.B. (1998). *Multisystemic Treatment of Antisocial Behavior in Children and Adolescents*. New York: Guilford Press.

Horner, G. (2010). Child Sexual Abuse: Consequences and Implications. *Journal of Pediatric Health Care*, 24, 358–364.

Karson, M. (2001). *Patterns of Child Abuse*. New York: Haworth.

Kaufman, K.L., Holmberg, J.K., Orts, K.A., McCrady, F.E., Rotsien, A.L., Daleiden, E.L., & Hilliker, D.R. (1998). Factors Influencing Sexual Offenders' Modus Operandi: An Examination of Victim-Offender Relatedness and Age. *Child Maltreatment*, 3, 349–361.

Kilpatrick, D.G. & Saunders, B.E. (1999). *Prevalence and Consequences of Child Victimization: Results from the National Survey of Adolescents (No. 93-IJ-CX-0023)*. Charleston, NC: National Crime Victims Research & Treatment Center, Department of Psychiatry, & Behavioral Sciences, Medical University of South Carolina.

Kinnally, E.L., Huang, Y., Haverly, R., Burke, A.K., Galfalvy, H., Brent, D.P, Oquendo, M.A., & Mann, J.J. (2009). Parental Care Moderates the Influence of MAOA-uVNTR Genotype and Childhood Stressors on Trait Impulsivity and Aggression in Adult Women. *Psychiatric Genetics*, 19, 126–133.

Kirsch, L.G., Fanniff, A.M., & Becker, J.V. (2011). Treatment of Adolescent and Adult Sexual Offenders. In J.E.B. Myers (Ed.), *The APSAC Handbook of Child Maltreatment*, 3rd edition, 289–305. Thousand Oaks, CA: Sage.

Lamb, M.E., Hershkowitz, I., Orbach, Y., & Esplin, P.W. (2008). *Tell Me What Happened: Structured Investigative Interviews of Child Victims and Witnesses*. London: Wiley.

Leifer, M., Shapiro, J.P., & Kassem, L. (1993). The Impact of Maternal History and Behavior Upon Foster Placement and Adjustment in Sexually Abused Girls. *Child Abuse and Neglect*, 17, 755–766.

Lev-Wiesel, R. (2008). Child Sexual Abuse: A Critical Review of Intervention and Treatment Modalities. *Children and Youth Services Review*, 3, 665–673.

Lock, J. (2009). Eating Disorders in Children and Adolescents. *Psychiatric Times*, 26, 35–38.

London, K., Bruck, M., Ceci, S.J., & Shuman, D.W. (2005). Disclosure of Child Sexual Abuse: What Does the Research Tell Us About the Ways That Children Tell? *Psychology, Public Policy, and Law*, 11, 194–226.

Lowe, K. & Pearce, J. (2006). Young People and Sexual Exploration. *Child Abuse Review*, 15, 289–293.

Lyon, T.D. (2002). Scientific Support for Expert Testimony on Child Sexual Abuse Accommodation. In J.R. Conte (Ed.), *Critical Issues in Child Sexual Abuse*, 107–138. Thousand Oaks, CA: Sage.

Lyon, T.D. (2009). Abuse Disclosure: What Adults Can Tell. In B.L. Bottoms, C.J. Najdowski, & G.S. Goodman (Eds.), *Children as Victims, Witnesses, and Offenders: Psychological Science and the Law*, 19–35. New York: Guilford Press.

Lyon, T.D. & Ahern, E.C. (2011). Disclosure of Child Sexual Abuse: Implications for Interviewing. In J.E.B. Myers (Ed.), *The APSAC Handbook on Child Maltreatment*, 3rd edition, 233–252. Thousand Oaks, CA: Sage.

Maniglio, R. (2009). The Impact of Child Sexual Abuse on Health: A Systematic Review of Reviews. *Clinical Psychology Review*, 29, 647–657.

Mannarino, A.P. & Cohen, J.A. (1997). Family-Related Variables and Psychological Symptom Formation in Sexually Abused Girls. *Journal of Child Sexual Abuse*, 5, 105–120.

Marshall, W.L. (1999). Current Status of North American Assessment and Treatment Programs for Sexual Offenders. *Journal of Interpersonal Violence*, 14, 221–239.

Mathews, R., Mathews, J., & Speltz, K. (1990). Female Sexual Offenders. In M. Hunter (Ed.), *The Sexually Abused Male*, vol. 1, 275–293. New York: Lexington Books.

McClain, N.M. & Garrity, S.E. (2011). Sex Trafficking and the Exploitation of Adolescents. *Journal of Obstetric, Gynecologic, & Neonatal Nursing*, 40, 243–252.

McCoy, M.L. & Keen, S.M. (2014). *Child Abuse and Neglect*, 2nd edition. New York: Psychology Press.

McGarth, R.J., Cumming, G.F., & Burchard, B.L. (2003). *Current Practices and Trends in Sexual Abuser Management: Safer Society 2002 Nationwide Survey*. Brandon, VT: Safer Society Press.

McLeer, S.V., Dixon, J.F., Henry, D., Ruggiero, K., Escovitz, K., Niedda, T., & Scholle, R. (1998). Psychopathology in Non-Clinically Referred Sexually Abused Children. *Journal of the American Academy of Child and Adolescent Psychiatry*, 37, 1326–1333.

Mitchell, K.J., Jones, L.M., Finkelhor, D., & Wolak, J. (2011). Internet-Facilitated Commercial Sexual Exploration of Children: Findings from a Nationally Representative Sample of Law Enforcement Agencies in the United States. *Sexual Abuse: A Journal of Research and Treatment*, 23 (1), 43–71.

Moran, P.B., Vucinich, S., & Hall, N.K. (2004). Associations Between Types of Maltreatment and Substance Use During Adolescence. *Child Abuse and Neglect*, 28, 565–574.

Noll, J.G., Shenk, C.E., & Putnam, K.T. (2009). Childhood Sexual Abuse and Adolescent Pregnancy: A Meta-Analytic Update. *Journal of Pediatric Psychology*, 34, 366–378.

Ogilvie, B. (2004). *Mother-Daughter Incest*. New York: Haworth.

Paine, M.L. & Hansen, D.J. (2002). Factors Influencing Children to Self-Disclose Sexual Abuse. *Clinical Psychology Review*, 22, 271–295.

Paolucci, E.O., Genuis, M.L., & Violato, C. (2001). A Meta-Analysis of the Published Research on the Effects of Child Sexual Abuse. *The Journal of Psychology*, 135 (1), 17–36.

Putnam, F.W. (2003). Ten-Year Research Update Review: Child Sexual Abuse. *Journal of the American Academy of Child and Adolescent Psychiatry*, 42, 269–278.

Rice, M.E. & Harris, G.T. (2003). What We Know and Don't Know About Treating Adult Sexual Offenders. In B.J. Winick & J.Q. LaFond (Eds.), *Protecting Society from Sexually Dangerous Offenders: Law, Justice, and Therapy*, 101–117. Washington, DC: American Psychological Association.

Rich, P. (2006). *Attachment and Sexual Offending*. West Sussex, UK: John Wiley and Sons.

Ruggiero, K.J., McLeer, S.V., & Dixon, J.F. (2000). Sexual Abuse Characteristics Associated with Survivor Psychopathology. *Child Abuse and Neglect*, 24, 951–964.

Sapp, M.V. & Vandeven, A.M. (2005). Update on Childhood Sexual Abuse. *Current Opinion in Pediatrics*, 17, 258–264.

Saunders, B.E., Kilpatrick, D.G., Hanson, R.F., Resnik, H.S., & Walker, M.E. (1999). Prevalence, Case Characteristics, and Long-Term Psychological Correlates of Child Rape Among Women: A National Survey. *Child Maltreatment*, 4, 187–200.

Sedlak, A.J., Mettenburg, J, Basena, M., Petta, I., McPherson, K., Greene, A., & Li, S. (2010). *Fourth Incidence Study of Child Abuse and Neglect (NIS-4): Report to Congress.* Washington, DC: US Department of Health and Human Services, Administration for Children and Families.

Shannon, D. (2008). Online Sexual Grooming in Sweden – Online Offences against Children as Described in Swedish Police Data. *Journal of Scandinavian Studies in Criminology and Crime Prevention*, 9, 160–180.

Sheinberg, M. & Fraenkel, P. (2001). *The Relational Trauma of Incest: A Family-Based Approach to Treatment.* New York: Guilford Press.

Shin, S.H., Hong, H.G., & Hazen, A.L. (2010). Childhood Sexual Abuse and Adolescent Substance Use: A Latent Class Analysis. *Drug and Alcohol Dependence*, 109 (1–3), 226–235. doi:10.1016/j.drugalcdep.2010.01.013.

Stein, T. (1998). *Child Welfare and the Law.* New York: Longman.

Sternberg, K.J., Lamb, M.E., Orbach, Y., Esplin, P.W., & Mitchell, S. (2001). Use of a Structured Investigative Protocol Enhances Young Children's Responses to Free Recall Prompts in the Course of Forensic Interviews. *Journal of Applied Psychology*, 86, 997–1005.

Tjaden, P. & Thoennes, N. (2000). *Full Report of the Prevalence, Incidence, and Consequences of Violence Against Women: Findings from the National Violence Against Women Survey.* Washington, DC: US Department of Justice, Office of Justice Programs, NCJ 183781.

van der Kolk, B.A. (2005). Developmental Trauma Disorder. *Psychiatric Annals*, 35 (3), 401–408.

Van Gerko, K., Hughes, M.L., Hamill, M., & Waller, G. (2005). Reported Childhood Sexual Abuse and Eating Disordered Cognitions and Behaviors. *Child Abuse and Neglect*, 29, 375–382.

van Roode, T., Dickson, N., Herbison, P., & Paul, C. (2009). Child Sexual Abuse and Persistence of Risky Sexual Behaviors and Negative Sexual Outcomes Over Adulthood: Findings from a Birth Cohort. *Child Abuse and Neglect*, 33, 161–172.

Webb, N.B. (1999). Play Therapy Crisis Intervention with Children. In N.B. Webb (Ed.), *Play Therapy with Children in Crisis*, 29–46. New York: Guilford Press.

Wickham, R.E. & West, J. (2003). *Therapeutic Work with Sexually Abused Children.* Thousand Oaks, CA: Sage.

Wiehe, V.R. (1997). *Sibling Abuse: Hidden Physical, Emotional, and Sexual Trauma.* Thousand Oaks, CA: Sage.

Wonderlich, S.A., Crosby, R.D., Mitchell, J.E., Roberts, J.A., Haseltine, B., DeMuth, G., & Thompson, K.M. (2000). Relationship of Childhood Sexual Abuse and Eating Disturbances in Children. *Journal of the American Academy of Child and Adolescent Psychiatry*, 39, 1277–1283.

Part III

Response to Child Maltreatment

9 The Child Protection Process

Identification of Maltreatment Victims

The first step of any response to child maltreatment is identification of the victim. Most states have mandated reporting laws, which require professionals, and sometimes citizens, to report incidents of child abuse and neglect. Mandated reporting is discussed in detail in Chapter 11.

Intake

Intake begins when the child protection agency receives a report of suspected abuse or neglect. Typically, these agencies are state- or county-run, and in some states can include the police department. When a report is received, two decisions must be made: (1) Does the report meet the guidelines of child abuse or neglect? and (2) How urgent is the report? These questions can be answered by the intake worker, who determines the following:

1 Was sufficient information provided in the report?
2 Does the accusation meet state or federal laws for abuse or neglect?
3 Is the reporter credible?
4 What type of maltreatment occurred?
5 What is the severity of harm to the child?
6 What is the relationship of the child to the perpetrator?
7 Does the perpetrator have access to the child? (Is the child safe?)
8 What is the child's vulnerability (age, illness, disability)?
9 Are there any other known cases of abuse or neglect by the perpetrator?
10 Who is available to protect the child?

(Goldman et al., 2003)

If all of these questions are answered sufficiently, the report is accepted and given to a child protection investigator. In most cases, the investigator is a person trained in child welfare, like a social worker. In some states, the

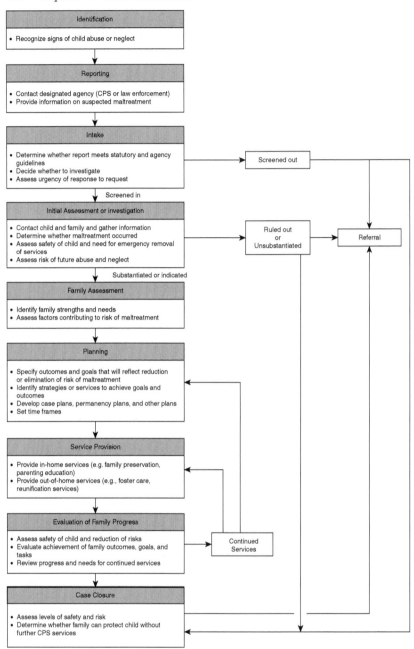

Figure 9.1 Overview of the Child Protection Process
Source: Adapted from Goldman et al., 2003, p. 60

investigator is a police officer or a team consisting of a child welfare worker and a police officer. If questions in the report cannot be answered, or if the accusation does not meet state or federal guidelines for abuse or neglect, the case is closed. In some instances, the case can be accepted even with limited information. In this case, the agency might conduct an investigation and offer the family voluntary services. An example of this type of case could be a family in poverty who cannot afford to buy lice treatment for their child. A school might report this as neglect because the child is continually sent to school with head lice and infects other children. The child protection agency can accept the report, offer voluntary services to the family in the form of monetary support to buy lice treatment, teach the family how to treat the child for lice, and then close the case. In this instance, the court system is not involved. The family must voluntarily agree to be involved in the child protection agency services, and the child's lice problem is treated.

Regardless of the outcome of a report of maltreatment, every state keeps an electronic record of the report, including the name of the victim and perpetrator. This information is an important record that can be used to show patterns of maltreatment and provide historical information about a perpetrator. Any person working with children, such as social workers, teachers, doctors, and others, who undergoes background screening for employment will be checked for child maltreatment reports.

Initial Investigation

Any report that is determined to meet the criteria for abuse or neglect receives an investigation. The child protection investigation reviews some of the questions asked during intake, such as:

- Does the allegation meet state or federal law for abuse or neglect?
- Is the child safe or at risk for more maltreatment?
- What is the level of risk, if the child is not safe?
- What type of intervention will ensure safety in the least intrusive manner?
- What type and what level of care does the child need if they are not safe?
- Does the family have needs that must be met?
- Does the family need services to reduce the risk of further maltreatment?

(DePanfilis & Salus, 2003; Goldman et al., 2003)

Child abuse and neglect investigations occur when a parent is accused of abuse or neglect. The same process is also used when other caregivers, such as childcare workers, teachers, or out-of-home care facilities are accused of abusing a child.

During this assessment period, other professionals may be involved to assist in determining the answers to the investigative questions. Medical personnel, such as nurses and doctors, may be involved to evaluate and determine if abuse or neglect occurred or to care for medical needs or injuries the child sustained. Mental health providers may be involved to determine if maltreatment occurred or to assess the effects of the maltreatment. Teachers or childcare providers are involved to provide information about the child and family and to provide support to the child during the investigation. Foster homes and other types of placement agencies are involved if a child needs to be removed from the family home and placed in out-of-home care.

After a complete investigation of the report has been completed, the child protection investigator must make a determination about the report. There are typically three types of investigative determinations:

1   **Substantiated**. A conclusion that there are allegations of abuse or neglect based on state or federal laws. This is the highest level of determination. At this point, the court system becomes involved and the case is referred to an ongoing child welfare worker who works closely with the child and the family.

2   **Indicated or Reason to Suspect Abuse or Neglect**. This determination indicates that abuse or neglect cannot be substantiated according to state or federal law, but the child may have been maltreated or is at risk for future maltreatment. Not all states have this determination. At this point, several things could occur. As described above, the family may be offered voluntary services, and the court system does not get involved. This allows the child protection agency to remain involved with the family and monitor for indications or further instances of maltreatment. In some cases, the court may be involved and order the family to work with the child protection agency to ensure the child remains safe. In both instances, the child would remain in the home under the care of the family with supervision from the child protection agency.

3   **Not Substantiated**. This determines that there is not sufficient evidence under state or federal law to conclude the child was maltreated or is at risk of future harm. At this point, the case is closed, but the record remains in the state system.

Risk or Safety Assessment

A risk or safety assessment is a decision-making process that evaluates the risk of harm to a child from maltreatment. This process is used to inform case decisions or modify family case plans. Risk assessment is an ongoing process throughout the case and is based on current information about the child and family (DePanfilis, 2005). Level of risk can change depending on risk and protective factors that are present at the time of assessment. In addition to specific risk or protective factors, the degree of risk is an important consideration. The presence of one protective factor may reduce a higher degree of risk to a low risk situation. Family information continually changes and must be factored into regular monitoring and evaluation of a case. Child welfare workers must be proficient in the assessment process so they can make the best decisions about a case. It is not enough to just use a tool or just rely on intuition to make decisions about risk or safety, according to Pecora, Chahine, and Graham (2013). Child welfare caseworkers must use both to make the best decisions. Brown and Packard (2012) completed a review of child welfare risk assessment instruments and found that three specific risk assessment tools were commonly used across the United States in child welfare agencies: Structured Decision Making® (SDM), Comprehensive Assessment Tool (CAT), and Signs of Safety (SOS). Because there are a variety of ways in which to assess risk, it is important to review one's own state requirements and to be a competent assessor and decision-maker.

Family Assessment

After an investigation determines a report is substantiated, the court system becomes involved. When the judge determines that the investigator is correct and maltreatment is substantiated, a court case is opened, and a child welfare caseworker is assigned to begin working with the child and the family. The start of this ongoing work with the child and family begins with an assessment. The assessment process is used to identify, consider, and weigh factors that affect the child's safety, permanency, and well-being as well as gain understanding of the family's strengths, needs, and resources (DePanfilis & Salus, 2003; Goldman et al., 2003).

Goldman, Salus, Wolkott, and Kennedy (2003), indicate that several key decisions are made as a result of the family assessment:

1 What are the *risks* and needs of this family that affect safety, permanency, or well-being?
2 What are the *effects* of maltreatment that affect safety, permanency, or well-being?
3 What are the individual and family *strengths*?
4 How do the *family members perceive* their conditions, problems, and strengths?
5 *What must change* in order for the effects of maltreatment to be addressed and risk to be reduced/eliminated?
6 What is the *parent's level of readiness* for change? What is the parent's motivation and capacity to assure safety, permanency, and well-being?
(Goldman et al., 2003, p. 69)

All assessments should be strengths-based and culturally sensitive (DePanfilis & Salus, 2003). The assessment process is a key time where the skill of the child welfare worker and their ability to establish a respectful working relationship with the family can impact the outcome of the case.

Types of Assessment

There are many tools available to assess child physical abuse, sexual abuse, or parenting ability. However, child neglect is the most frequently occurring type of maltreatment in the United States and internationally. In 2009, more than 75% of child maltreatment cases in the United States were classified as neglect (Children's Bureau & NCANDS, 2010). Additionally, England, Ireland, and Australia report similar findings (see, for example, Campbell, 1997; Dickens, 2006; Jones & Gupta 1998; McSherry, 2007; Stone, 2007). Bundy-Fazioli & DeLong Hamilton (2010) provide a multi-dimensional framework for assessment (Table 9.1) that was developed using systems theory and the belief that individuals exist in a reciprocal relationship with their environment (Payne, 2005). The assessment framework has three areas including strengths and challenges, parent's perception and awareness, and agency involvement. The multi-dimensional framework provides a guideline for child welfare workers to focus on family strengths and encourages communication between the worker and family (Bundy-Fazioli & DeLong Hamilton, 2010). Although this assessment was developed specifically for cases of neglect, its comprehensive nature makes it useful for assessing of all types of child maltreatment (see Table 9.1).

Case Planning

Upon completion of a comprehensive assessment of the child and family, the child welfare worker and family work together to complete a case plan. The case planning process varies but is based on the completed assessment. Case plans should be strengths-based, culturally sensitive, and developed with the family (DePanfilis & Salus, 2003). The team approach in case planning can include extended family and other supportive individuals. This approach is referred to as team decision-making. Whatever approach is taken to case planning, it is crucial to develop the plan with the family. The team approach ensures the family's commitment to completing the case plan, and it empowers them to change (DePanfilis & Salus, 2003; Goldman et al., 2003).

Case plans may look different across agencies and states, but all have similar content, which includes outcomes, measurable goals, interventions or services, and time frames for completion of tasks. The court is appraised of the case plan and monitors family progress along with the child welfare worker. Monitoring and completion of the case plan in a timely manner ensures that children and families do not linger in the child welfare system for an unnecessary amount of time.

Table 9.1 Multi-Dimensional Framework for Assessment

Areas of Strengths & Challenges	Parents' Perception and Awareness			Agency Involvement	
	History Pattern	Change beyond PC*	Change within PC*	Current	Past
Parent History					
Significant Events					
Child History					
Developmental Milestones					
Parent Well-being					
■ Mental health status					
■ Substance use & abuse					
■ Domestic violence					
■ Trauma, grief, loss					
■ Communication skills					
■ Physical health					
■ Education learning					
Child Well-being					
■ Mental health Status					
■ Substance use & abuse					
■ Type of neglect/abuse					
■ Trauma, grief, loss					
■ Friends & activities					
■ Physical health					
■ Education learning					
Parent-Child/Family Well-being					
■ Familial Status (who lives in the home?)					
■ Basic needs (housing, food, clothes)					
■ Parenting skills (discipline, attachment, safety, basic needs, protection, values)					
■ Parent-child interaction					
■ Child interaction with relatives					
Community/ Environmental					
■ Housing					
■ Neighborhood					

(continued)

Areas of Strengths & Challenges	Parents' Perception and Awareness			Agency Involvement	
	History Pattern	*Change beyond PC★*	*Change within PC★*	*Current*	*Past*
■ Child/family activities (church, school, etc)					
■ Transportration					
Social Supports					
■ Friends					
■ Family					
■ Job					
Financial Supports					
■ Employment					

Concurrent Planning or Differential Response

After a full assessment of the family is completed, some child welfare agencies also complete a differential response plan. A differential response is a back-up plan in case the family cannot complete the case plan (CWIG, 2011). The Child Abuse Prevention and Treatment Act of 2020 (2010) requires all states to refer children who are "not at risk of imminent harm to a community organization or voluntary preventive service" (p. 19). A differential response plan is used for families with low to moderate risk of abuse and neglect and allows child protection agencies more flexibility to intervene (Karter & Daro, 2016). Researchers have found that differential response plans are often associated with increased services for the family, fewer subsequent reports of abuse and neglect, fewer re-assessments, and fewer removals from the family home (Lawrence et al., 2011; Loman et al., 2010; Loman & Siegel, 2004; Siegel et al., 2010; Winokur et al., 2015). With a differential response plan in place, the child and family receive consistent assessment and evaluation from the child welfare worker, which ensures appropriate services are in place to support the family and keep the child safe.

Family Services

After the case plan has been developed and approved, the child welfare worker makes referrals for all services identified in the case plan. The services are an important component of the case because they help the family achieve their case plan goals (Goldman et al., 2003). Each type of service should support the goals and be tailored for the family's specific needs. Making the mistake of referring every family on a caseload to the same services is a cookie-cutter approach that does not support and ensure a successful case outcome. In-home services work well for families who have minimal safety issues. Agency-based services are best for families who have had a child removed due to safety issues or higher risk or safety situations.

Monitoring and Evaluation

Evaluation of the case is a continual process that starts from the beginning and continues until case closure. Child welfare workers have mandated contact with children and families, usually on a monthly basis. During each visit, the worker should assess the progress the family is making and complete a risk assessment to determine child safety (DePanfilis & Salus, 2003). Court reviews of cases occur about every three months until the case closes. Goldman, Salus, Wolkott, and Kennedy (2003) suggest eight questions to assist with the monitoring and evaluation process:

1   Is the child safe? Have the protective factors, strengths, or the safety factors changed, warranting a change or elimination of the safety plan or the development of a safety plan?
2   What changes, if any, have occurred with respect to the conditions and behaviors contributing to the risk of maltreatment?
3   What outcomes have been accomplished, and how does the worker know that they have been accomplished?
4   What progress has been made toward achieving case goals?
5   Have the services been effective in helping clients achieve outcomes and goals and, if not, what adjustments need to be made to improve outcomes?
6   What is the current level of risk in the family?
7   Have the risk factors been reduced sufficiently so that parents can protect the children and meet their developmental needs so that the case can be closed?
8   Has it been determined that reunification is not likely and there is no significant progress toward outcomes? If so, is an alternative plan needed?

(Goldman et al., 2003, pp. 71–2)

Case Closure

A judge is the only person who can officially close a child welfare case. This happens upon the recommendation of the child welfare caseworker who has been working closely with the family and monitoring progress on case plan completion. Case closure recommendations can stem from successful completion of a case or unsuccessful completion of a case. In successful instances, the family may have completed their case plan or have been referred to another agency. In unsuccessful instances, termination of parental rights can occur. Cases can also close if the family discontinues contact with the child welfare agency. Unfortunately, if a family moves to another state, agency computer systems are not linked and do not have the ability to communicate about shared clients. If a family decides to move when an open child welfare case exists, nothing can be done except alert the state the family moved to or hope the family takes it upon themselves to seek assistance and complete the plan that was started.

It is important to follow a process for case closure according to DePanfilis and Salus (2003). This process includes meeting with the family and reviewing risk reduction, reviewing completed tasks, reviewing general steps for problem solving, and considering any remaining needs or concerns the family may have.

References

Brown, K. & Packard, T. (2012). *Review of Child Welfare Risk Assessments: Southern Area Consortium of Human Services.* San Diego, CA: Academy for Professional Excellence at San Diego State University School of Social Work.

Bundy-Fazioli, K. & DeLong Hamilton, T.A. (2010). Educating Social Workers on Child Neglect: A Multi-Dimensional Framework. *Professional Development: The International Journal of Continuing Social Work Education,* 13 (1), 40–46.

Campbell, L. (1997). Child Neglect and Intensive Family-Preservation Practice. *Families in Society,* 78 (3), 280–290.

Child Abuse Prevention and Treatment Act of 2010 (2010). Public Law 111–320, December 12.

Children's Bureau & NCANDS. (2010). *Child Maltreatment 2009.* Washington, DC: US Department of Health and Human Services, Administration for Children and Families, Administration on Children, Youth and Families, Children's Bureau. Retrieved from: http://www.acf.hhs.gov/programs/cb/stats_research/index.htm#can.

CWIG (Child Welfare Information Gateway). (2011). *Child Maltreatment Prevention: Past, Present, and Future.* Washington, DC: US Department of Health and Human Services, Children's Bureau.

DePanfilis, D. (2005). Child Protection. In G.P. Mallon & P.M. Hess (Eds.), *Child Welfare for the 21st Century: A Handbook of Practices, Policies, and Programs,* 290–301. New York: Columbia University Press.

DePanfilis, D. & Salus, M.K. (2003). *Child Protective Services: A Guide for Caseworkers.* Washington, DC: US Department of Health and Human Services Administration for Children and Families Administration on Children, Youth and Families Children's Bureau Office on Child Abuse and Neglect.

Dickens, J. (2006). Child Neglect and the Law: Catapults, Thresholds, and Delays. *Child Abuse Review,* 16, 77–92.

Goldman, J., Salus, M.K., Wolkott, D., & Kennedy, K.Y. (2003). *A Coordinated Response to Child Abuse and Neglect: The Foundation for Practice.* Washington, DC: US Department of Health and Human Services, Administration for Children and Families, Administration on Children, Youth, and Families, Children's Bureau, Office on Child Abuse and Neglect.

Jones, J. & Gupta, A. (1998). The Context of Decision-Making in Cases of Child Neglect. *Child Abuse & Neglect*, 26, 679–695.

Karter, C. & Daro, D. (2016). *Planning to Prevent Child Maltreatment: Strategies to Support an Integrated Child Maltreatment Prevention Framework*. Chicago, IL: Chapin Hall at the University of Chicago.

Lawrence, C.N., Rosanbalm, K.D., & Dodge, K.A. (2011). Multiple Response System: Evaluation of Policy Change in North Carolina's Child Welfare System. *Children & Youth Services Review*, 33 (11), 2355–2365.

Loman, L.A., Filonow, C.S., & Siegel, G. (2010). *Ohio Alternative Response Evaluation: Final Report*. St. Louis, MO: Institute of Applied Research.

Loman, L.A. & Siegel, G.L. (2004). *Minnesota Alternative Response Evaluation: Final Report*. St. Louis, MO: Institute of Applied Research.

McSherry, D. (2007). Understanding and Addressing the "Neglect of Neglect": Why Are We Making a Mole-Hill Out of a Mountain? *Child Abuse & Neglect*, 31, 607–614.

Payne, M. (2005). *Modern Social Work Theory*, 2nd edition. Chicago, IL: Lyceum Books, Inc.

Pecora, P.J., Chahine, Z., & Graham, J.C. (2013). Safety and Risk Assessment Frameworks: Overview and Implications for Child Maltreatment Fatalities. *Child Welfare*, 92 (2), 143–160.

Siegel, G.L., Filonow, C.S., & Loman, L.A. (2010). *Differential Response in Nevada: Final Evaluation Report*. St. Louis: MO: Institute of Applied Research.

Stone, S. (2007). Child Maltreatment, Out-of-Home Placement and Academic Vulnerability: A Fifteen-Year Review of Evidence and Future Directions. *Children and Youth Services Review*, 29, 139–161.

Winokur, M., Ellis, R., Drury, I., & Rogers, J. (2015). Answering the Big Questions About Differential Response in Colorado: Safety and Cost Outcomes from a Randomized Controlled Trial. *Child Abuse & Neglect*, 39, 98–108.

10 Professional Considerations

Philosophy of Child Protective Services

Similar to theories that guide our practice, there is also a philosophy that most child protective services workers adhere to in order to ensure their practice is ethical and child-focused. DePanfilis and Salus (2003), provide the following philosophy about child protective services:

- A safe and permanent home and family is the best place for a child to grow up.
- Most parents want to be good parents and, when adequately supported, they have the strength and capacity to care for their children and keep them safe.
- Families who need assistance from a child protection agency are diverse in terms of structure, culture, race, religion, economic status, beliefs, values, and lifestyles.
- Child protection agencies are held accountable for achieving outcomes of child safety, permanence, and family well-being.
- Child protection efforts are most likely to succeed when clients are involved and actively participate in the process.
- When parents cannot or will not fulfill their responsibilities to protect their children, child protection has the right and obligation to intervene directly on the children's behalf.
- When children are placed in out-of-home care because their safety cannot be assured, child protection should develop a permanency plan as soon as possible.
- To best protect a child's overall well-being, agencies want to assure that children move to permanency as quickly as possible.

Goldman, Salus, Wolkott, and Kennedy (2003) created specific tenets based on federal child protection laws and commonly held values and beliefs about parenting. United States federal law tells us that parents have a right to raise their children according to their own values and beliefs, but when those values or beliefs are unhealthy or abusive, state governments have the right to step in and protect children from harm. The philosophical tenets below, explained by Goldman, Salus, Wolkott, and Kennedy (2003), are the principles discussed in the Adoption and Safe Families Act.

1 **Prevention programs are necessary to strengthen families and reduce the likelihood of child abuse and neglect.** Child maltreatment results from a combination of factors: psychological, social, situational, and societal. Factors that may contribute to an increased risk for child abuse and neglect include, for example, family structure, poverty, substance abuse, poor housing conditions, teenage pregnancy, domestic and community violence, mental illness, and lack of support from extended families and community members. To reduce the occurrence of maltreatment, communities should develop and implement prevention programs that support children and families.

2 **The responsibility for addressing child maltreatment is shared among community professionals and citizens.** No single agency, individual, or discipline has all the necessary knowledge, skills, or resources to provide the assistance needed by abused and neglected children and their families. While public child protective services (CPS) agencies, law enforcement, and courts have legal mandates and primary responsibility for responding to child maltreatment, other service providers working with children and families—along with community members—play important roles in supporting families and protecting children. To be effective in addressing this complex problem, the combined expertise and resources of interdisciplinary agencies and professionals are needed.

3 **A safe and permanent home is the best place for a child to grow up.** Most children are best cared for in their own families. Children naturally develop a strong attachment to their families and when removed from them, they typically experience loss, confusion, and other negative emotions. Maintaining the family as a unit preserves important relationships with parents, siblings, and extended family members and allows children to grow and develop within their own culture and environment.

4 **When parents (or caregivers) are unable or unwilling to fulfill their responsibilities to provide adequate care and to keep their children safe, CPS has the mandate to intervene.** Both laws and good practice maintain that interventions should be designed to help parents protect their children in the least intrusive manner possible. Interventions should build on the family's strengths and address the factors that contribute to the risk of maltreatment. Reasonable efforts must be made to maintain child safety and keep the children with their families except when there is significant risk to child safety. Referral to court and removal of children from their families should only be done when it is determined that children cannot be kept safely in their own homes.

5 **Most parents want to be good parents and have the strength and capacity, when adequately supported, to care for their children and keep them safe.** Underlying CPS intervention is the belief that people have the strength and potential to change their lives. Professionals must search for and identify the strengths and the inner resiliencies in families that provide the foundation for change.

6 **To help families protect their children and meet their basic needs, the community's response must demonstrate respect for every person involved.** All people deserve to be treated with respect and dignity. This means showing respect for a person, while not necessarily approving or condoning his or her actions. In addition to caregivers and children, service providers should demonstrate respect for mothers, fathers, grandparents, other family members, and the family's support network.

7 **Services must be individualized and tailored.** While people may have similar problems, there are elements that will vary from family to family. In addition, each family's strengths and resources are different. The community's response, therefore, must be customized to reflect the particular circumstances, strengths, and needs of each family.

8 **Child protection and service delivery approaches should be family centered.** Parents, children, their extended families, and support networks (e.g., the faith community, teachers, health care providers, substitute caregivers) should be actively involved as partners in developing and implementing appropriate plans and services to reduce or eliminate the risk of maltreatment. Tapping into the strengths and resources of a family's natural support network is fundamental to enhancing family functioning.

9 **Interventions need to be sensitive to the cultures, beliefs, and customs of all families.** Professionals must acknowledge and show respect for the values and traditions of families from diverse cultural, ethnic, and religious backgrounds. To become culturally competent, professionals must first understand themselves and the effects of their own background on their values, behaviors, and judgments about others. In working with children and families different from themselves, professionals need to be aware of the context of the family's culture and background in order to help provide access to culturally relevant services and solutions.

10 **To best protect a child's overall well-being, agencies must assure that children move to permanency as quickly as possible.** Along with developing plans to facilitate reunification of children, agencies must develop alternative plans for permanence from the time the child enters care. For those children who cannot be safely reunified with their families, timely efforts must be made to ensure a stable, secure, and permanent home for the child through adoption or other permanent living arrangements.

(Goldman et al., 2003, pp. 10–11)

Children's Rights vs. Parents' Rights

In addition to the guiding theories and philosophies in child welfare practice, it is important to be able to distinguish between children's right and parents' rights. Children have the right to live in healthy, non-abusive environments with parents who ensure their basic needs are being met. Children have the right to grow up in a permanent family and the right to legal representation during court activities to ensure their best interests.

Understanding the difference between parent and child rights is one of the primary, ethical dilemmas that social workers in child welfare face. Often, when child welfare workers advocate for the rights of the children on their caseloads, it can cause conflict with parents and parents' rights to raise children as they see fit. As a child welfare worker, it is important to base decisions about children and their parents on facts to ensure the rights of both are at the forefront. At the same time, a child welfare worker's own values or beliefs should be kept out of the decision-making process. To ensure decisions are made in the most ethical manner as possible, the child welfare worker must be familiar with federal and state laws; knowledgeable about parenting, child development, and children's and parents' rights; and use an ethical decision-making model.

Caseworker Competence: Knowledge, Values, and Skills

DePanfilis and Salus (2003) created a list of core values, knowledge, and skills that all social workers should have when working in the child welfare field, which includes understanding family systems, human growth and development, child abuse and neglect dynamics, cultural diversity, the continuum of placement services, and services available for children and families (DePanfilis & Salus, 2003).

The core values include the "belief that all people have the ability to facilitate change, every child has the right to grow up in a permanent family, and every child and family should be empowered to meet their own needs and goals" (DePanfilis & Salus, 2003, p. 12). To support these core values, social workers use strength-based practices, assure children are safe, practice confidentiality, set goals and ensure accountability, engage in quality social work practice, and continually work on increasing knowledge and skills to be an effective practitioner (DePanfilis & Salus, 2003).

The core skills that every child welfare worker should have include the ability to:

> identify strengths and needs and engage the family in a strength-based assessment process; take decisive and appropriate action when a child needs protection; analyze complex information; be persistent in approach to CPS work; employ crisis intervention and early intervention services and strategies; assess a family's readiness to change and

employ appropriate strategies for increasing motivation and building the helping alliance; function as a case manager and a team member, and collaborate with other service providers; assess for substance abuse, domestic violence, sexual abuse, and mental illness; [and] work with birth families to create a permanent plan for a child in foster care, kinship care, or group care.

(DePanfilis & Salus, 2003, p. 14)

In addition, social workers should be able to develop and maintain professional relationships with families; listen; be flexible; work with involuntary clients; work with legal systems; empower children and their families; assess for abuse, neglect, and safety; negotiate, implement and evaluate a case plan; work with service providers and supports; and apply knowledge of human behavior and intervention (Chang et al., 2018; DePanfilis & Salus, 2003).

The Role and Responsibilities of Child Welfare Workers

The basic role of the child welfare worker is to manage cases, engage in regular visits with the child and the family, conduct ongoing assessments and evaluate progress, attend team meetings to review cases, provide reports and attend court hearings, and provide ongoing referrals to supportive services. In addition to the basic responsibilities of the job, all child welfare workers are responsible for engaging in professional relationships with the clients on their caseloads (both children and parents). This includes the ability to communicate effectively and non-judgmentally and display empathy, respect, and genuineness.

Empathy is the ability to understand the feelings and experiences of another individual and then communicate compassion for those feelings and experiences (Chang et al., 2018; DePanfilis & Salus, 2003). Empathy builds trust and rapport in a relationship and can be displayed by "paying attention to verbal and nonverbal cues; communicating an understanding of the children's and family's message; showing a desire to understand; discussing what is important to the children and family; and referring to the children's and family's feelings" (DePanfilis & Salus, 2003, p. 18).

Respect is the ability to accept and value another individual and communicate this through caring behavior and communication (Chang et al., 2018; DePanfilis & Salus, 2003). For example, respect is demonstrated through engaging in culturally competent practices.

Genuineness means being yourself and incorporating your own personality into your professional role as a child welfare worker (Chang et al., 2018; DePanfilis & Salus, 2003). Child welfare workers are genuine when they do not take on a role or act fake, ensure nonverbal and verbal responses match, use eye contact and other nonverbal behaviors to communicate acceptance, express feelings appropriately without being artificial, and engage in non-defensive behavior (DePanfilis & Salus, 2003).

Supervision

Supervision is key to ensuring ethical and appropriate child welfare practice. Supervision can be in the form of formal or informal support. Formal support can be provided within an agency by experienced peers, supervisors, administrators, or an outside consultant. Supervision does not end after one has gained a number of years of experience. Supervision should be ongoing to ensure child welfare workers continue to engage in healthy, ethical, and appropriate practice within the NASW Code of Ethics. Supervision can include:

> communicating the agency's mission, policies, and practice guidelines to casework staff; setting standards of performance for staff to assure high-quality practice; assuring that all laws and policies are followed, and staying current with changing policies and procedures; creating a psychological and physical climate that enables staff to feel positive, satisfied, and comfortable about the job so that clients may be better served; helping staff learn what they need to know to effectively perform their jobs through orientation, mentoring, on-the-job training, and coaching; monitoring workloads and unit and staff performance to assure that standards and expectations are successfully achieved; keeping staff apprised of their performance and providing recognition for staff efforts and accomplishments; [and] implementing safety precautions"
>
> (DePanfilis & Salus, 2003, p. 105)

References

Chang, V., Decker, C., & Scott, S. (2018). *Developing Healing Skills: A Step-by-Step Approach to Competency*, 3rd edition. Boston, MA: Cengage.

DePanfilis, D. & Salus, M.K. (2003). *Child Protective Services: A Guide for Caseworkers*. Washington, DC: US Department of Health and Human Services Administration for Children and Families Administration on Children, Youth and Families Children's Bureau Office on Child Abuse and Neglect.

Goldman, J., Salus, M.K., Wolkott, D., & Kennedy, K.Y. (2003). *A Coordinated Response to Child Abuse and Neglect: The Foundation for Practice*. Washington, DC: US Department of Health and Human Services, Administration for Children and Families, Administration on Children, Youth, and Families, Children's Bureau, Office on Child Abuse and Neglect.

11 Mandated Reporting

What Is Mandated Reporting?

While all social work students throughout the United States learn early in their studies that they are mandated reporters of suspected child maltreatment, the role of mandated reporter has not existed throughout the development of our profession. Mandated reporting has only been in place for a little more than 50 years. After the 1962 Kempe et al. article on battered-child syndrome in the *Journal of the American Medical Association*, many policy proposals were offered in an effort to prevent child abuse and protect abused children from further harm.

In the early phases of child welfare policy development, a consistent recommendation was to mandate that physicians report child abuse. It was believed that if professionals who have contact with children and families, namely medical personnel, were required to report suspected child abuse, then the government could step in and protect children at risk before they were irreversibly harmed. The policy, referred to as "mandated reporting", was the first of its kind in the world.

Mandated reporting laws require certain people, mandated reporters, to make reports of suspected child maltreatment to a governmental authority. Failure to do so can trigger legal consequences against the mandated reporters. These laws also set up legal protections to encourage mandated reporters to fulfill their obligations.

As a result of large-scale efforts to institute mandated reporting laws, by 1967 all 50 states and the District of Columbia passed legislation requiring doctors and other medical personnel to report suspected child maltreatment. The new policy was considered a great success. In New York State, for instance, within five years of passing its first mandated reporting law, child fatalities dropped by 50% (Hutchison, 1993).

Who Are Mandated Reporters?

Mandated reporters are individuals required by the law of a given state to report concerning suspicions. Most often the term "mandated reporter" refers to individuals required to report suspicions of child abuse or neglect, but in some states the law may require certain people to report elder abuse, institutional corruption, etc. This chapter focuses on the role of mandated reporters of suspected child abuse and neglect.

Most state laws list adults with certain professional classifications as mandated reporters. Most often they are medical personnel, law enforcement, educational personnel, mental health professionals, social service workers, and social workers. Social workers are, in fact, mandated reporters in *all* 50 states.

On the other hand, 18 states and Puerto Rico have adopted laws that require *all adults*, regardless of occupation or professional classification, to report suspicions of child maltreatment. We refer to these states as "Universal Mandated Reporting" (UMR) states. As of 2016, the list of UMR states includes: Delaware, Florida, Idaho, Indiana, Kentucky, Maryland, Mississippi, Nebraska, New Hampshire, New Jersey, New Mexico, North Carolina, Oklahoma, Rhode Island, Tennessee, Texas, Utah, and Wyoming. The requirement to report in these states extends to suspicions that arise out of personal as well as professional observations. So, in Universal Mandated Reporting states, all adults are required to report suspicions, even if they relate to family members, friends, and/or acquaintances.

In the other 32 states, which list professional titles or roles that are deemed mandated reporters, most reports are only required when the child maltreatment suspicions arise from observations made in the professional role. In these states, if suspicions of child maltreatment develop outside the confines of an individual's professional obligations, then the law most likely does not legally require a report be made. There are state-specific laws on this issue, however, so always consult the law in your individual state.

It is important to note that, when there are differences in mandated reporting laws across states, you are legally obligated to follow the law of the state in which you are physically located. For instance, if you work in a Universal Mandated Reporting state but live in one of the other 32 states, you would be responsible for making reports outside your professional role if suspicions develop from observations made on your lunch break in the state where you work, but you would not be required to do so if your suspicions arise from similar observations in your home state.

Professionals, mostly mandated reporters, make more than half of the reports that CPS receives in a given year in the United States. In 2014, law enforcement personnel, namely the police, were the largest single source of reports, making 16% of all reports (US DHHS, Administration on Children, Youth, and Families, 2015). Educational personnel, namely teachers, made up the second largest single report source, submitting more than 15% of all reports (US DHHS, Administration on Children, Youth, and Families, 2015). The third largest source of reports are social services workers, who made more than 10% of all reports received by CPS in 2014 (US DHHS, Administration on Children, Youth, and Families, 2015).

Non-professionals (including alleged victims, their family members, neighbors, and anonymous tipsters) also make reports to CPS, though in most states they are *not* mandated reporters. Of non-professional sources, anonymous reporters make the most reports, almost 9% of the total number (US DHHS, Administration on Children, Youth, and Families, 2015). Although reports are received from professionals and non-professionals alike, professional reporters tend to have their reports substantiated at a higher rate than non-professional reporters.

How Do Social Workers Negotiate Conflicting Ethical and Legal Requirements as Mandated Reporters?

Since social workers work with children and families in a variety of settings and roles, it makes sense that laws in all 50 states require social workers to report suspicions of child abuse and neglect. Though some social work settings, like schools, hospitals, and mental health clinics, are more likely to yield suspicions of child maltreatment than others, like nursing homes, all social workers regardless of setting are mandated reporters of suspected child abuse and neglect.

Unlike many other types of mandated reporters, the social worker's role as mandated reporter needs to be considered in light of the ethical responsibilities of the profession. Guidance on ethical decision-making for social workers can be found in the Code of Ethics for the National Association of Social Workers (National Association of Social Workers, 2008). The latest version of the Code was revised in 2008. The Code provides that "social workers' primary goal is to help people in need and to address social problems" (National Association of Social Workers, 2008, Ethical Principle). By not reporting a case of suspected child abuse or neglect, the social worker fails to fulfill this ethical principle because the failure to report may subject the child to harm from abuse or neglect.

Social workers familiar with the NASW Code are aware of the sections that emphasize the importance of keeping client communications confidential. Therefore, social workers are often concerned that breaking the confidentiality of their relationship with a client to report suspected child abuse or neglect is a violation of the Code. However, the Code specifically provides that "social workers should protect the confidentiality of all information obtained in the course of professional service, *except for compelling professional reasons* [italics added]" (National Association of Social Workers, 2008, 1.07[c]). For instance, the expectation that social workers "keep information confidential does not apply when disclosure is necessary to prevent serious, foreseeable, an imminent harm to a client or other identifiable person" (National Association of Social Workers, 2008, 1.07[c]). This exception would include reporting suspicions of child abuse or neglect.

Even though the Code allows social workers to break client confidentiality for instances such as the mandated reporting of child abuse and neglect, the Code simultaneously highlights the importance of "disclosing the least amount of confidential information necessary to achieve the desired purpose" (National Association of Social Workers, 2008, 1.07[c]). When making a report to CPS, social workers should only provide information that is "directly relevant" to the suspicions and subsequent investigation. Social workers should protect all other client confidential information that is not relevant to the CPS report and investigation.

Social workers are subject to the same system developed to require mandated reporters to report suspicions of child maltreatment. However, due to the unique roles social workers play in the systems that clients interact with, it is important for social workers to be informed and aware of the context in which their reports are required.

How Does Mandated Reporting Work?

In order to fully understand how mandated reporting works, some background on how the policy developed is important. The first laws instituting systems of mandated reporting were designed at the state, not the federal, level. Starting in the mid-1960s, 50 different states authored legislation, producing a lot of variability across the country. These differences led to confusion and concern, because observations that required a report in one state did not necessarily require a report in a neighboring state. As was the practice during that particular period in US history, the federal government eventually stepped in to encourage uniformity through laws like the CAPTA of 1974 (see Chapter 3 for more detail on how the federal government encourages uniformity in child protection laws).

By 1980 most states passed the model child welfare legislation that was offered by the federal government. These laws expanded the definition of child abuse and neglect, offered a long list of professional titles to be identified as mandated reporters, and provided the legal measures for protecting and enforcing mandated reporting in the states. The adoption of these laws increased uniformity across states at the time. Subsequent changes in state laws over the next 30 years, however, again produced variability across states, though much less so than before the federal efforts of the 1970s.

At the advent of mandated reporting laws, mandated reporters in most states were required to make reports to the local police, juvenile courts, or the local social service agency. However, none of these government services was specifically designed to meet the needs of the child welfare system and many were severely understaffed.

Some policymakers wanted law enforcement to receive reports of suspected child abuse and conduct the resulting investigations. Many forms of child maltreatment were already under the purview of law enforcement, such as sexual abuse and severe physical abuse. The police were already staffed around the clock, every day of the year, so the infrastructure was already available. Additionally, American citizens were already accustomed to calling the police for help, so another system would not have to be learned. There was concern, however, that the police lacked the ability to provide therapeutic resources to afflicted families (Sussman & Cohen, 1975).

The juvenile courts at the time were deemed inappropriate to receive and investigate suspicions of child maltreatment. Since the courts ultimately decided the validity of allegations, it was believed that they should not also be responsible for the investigation (Sussman & Cohen, 1975). Additionally, the juvenile courts of the era were busy responding to numerous United States Supreme Court decisions, which were drastically changing their way of practice. For instance, the Court's decision in *In Re Gault* (1967) provided those accused of juvenile delinquency many rights previously denied to them, including the right to counsel and the right against self-incrimination.

At the time, the federal government decided that state-level departments of social services were the most appropriate venue for receiving and investigating reports of child maltreatment. Many states had already made this choice for themselves. It was also assumed that these departments would be best able to develop specialized offices for child protective services. These departments were expected to provide social service or treatment to families who needed intervention. The department of social services was seen as the non-punitive option. The goal was for reporters and families to see the department of social services as offering help and not just punishing wrongdoing. However, there was concern that, since departments of social service were already viewed as a "poor people's agency", child maltreatment may, as a result, be perceived as a problem exclusively of the poor (Sussman & Cohen, 1975). Today in most states child protection services and the mechanisms through which reports of suspected child maltreatment are received are generally still housed in departments of social services.

When mandated reporting laws were first adopted, reports of suspected child maltreatment were received and investigated at the local level. As a result, a family reported and investigated in one part of a state could simply move to another county, where the details of the prior investigation would not be available to the authorities. The laws aimed at encouraging uniformity across states also recommended the creation of a state central register to record all state reports. Central registers were designed to centralize data management in an effort to lessen the fiscal impact on county child protective services offices and improve the tracking of families involved in child welfare (Sussman & Cohen, 1975).

In many states, including New York, the state central register was designed to directly accept almost all reports from across the state. The central register then transmitted the information to the local child protective service agency, usually at the county level, to start an investigation. Using a central register to serve as a repository and receive reports streamlines the reporting process so that mandated reporters do not need access to multiple phone numbers to report maltreatment across county lines. Improvements in communication technologies over the past 50 years, from the advent of the facsimile ("fax") machine to the internet, have helped to speed up the transfer of information between state central registers and local county child protective offices.

When Do Mandated Reporters Have to Make a Report?

In most states, the law requires mandated reporters to make a call to child protective services as soon as they have *reasonable suspicion (or reasonable cause to suspect/believe)* that child abuse or neglect is occurring or is about to occur. Reasonable suspicion exists when a mandated reporter, based on training and experience in combination with what the individual observed/was told, entertains the possibility that a child is being abused and/or neglected or is in imminent danger of abuse or neglect. It may be enough that explanations provided by a parent and/or child were inconsistent with the observations, experience, and knowledge of the mandated reporter. Mandated reporters are not expected to be *sure* that child abuse or maltreatment has taken place, just reasonably suspicious (Lau et al., 2008).

A belief or suspicion is *reasonable* if someone else with similar education, training, and professional experience would have the same suspicion. Reasonable suspicion can start with the feeling that something does not feel right; however, a gut feeling without other concerns is not "reasonable". The mandated reporter is expected to objectively identify and examine any potential biases and overcome those that might interfere with the reporter's ability to be reasonable. Supervision and consultation with supervisors and colleagues can help.

If a mandated reporter consults with a supervisor or colleague and there is agreement that the suspicions warrant a report to CPS, the "reasonable suspicion" standard has been met. However, if the supervisor or colleague does not share the mandated reporter's suspicions, then the mandated reporter may not have reasonable suspicion. For instance, if the supervisor or colleague points out that the mandated reporter may be processing suspicions through personal biases, then the mandated reporter does not have reasonable suspicion. If, based on consultation, the mandated reporter no longer feels suspicious, then a report is not required. However, if the mandated reporter disagrees with the assessment of the supervisor or colleague and continues to believe that her/his suspicions are valid, then a report is still required by law.

While making the decision to report suspected child maltreatment is never an easy one, the legal standard of reasonable suspicion puts a very low burden of proof on the mandated reporter. This standard was designed to encourage reports of suspicions, instead of discouraging them. It follows from the idea that it is better to err on the side of protecting children.

What Protections Exist for Mandated Reporters?

The drafters of original mandated reporting legislation were aware that, unless there were incentives and protections for mandated reporters, everyone, whether required by law or not, would be hesitant to make reports of suspected child maltreatment, especially if they were not confident in their suspicions. Many reporters wonder, What if I'm wrong? Can I be sued? Can I lose my license? These are all important questions. To address these concerns, federal law requires states to protect reporters from legal action when fulfilling their legal obligation to report. In order to receive federal grants for their child protective system, states must include an immunity provision in their laws to protect mandated reporters (Child Abuse Prevention and Treatment Act, 1974).

If the resulting investigation does, in fact, substantiate the allegations raised by a reporter, mandated or not, there is no possible legal action against the reporter. However, if the resulting investigation does not substantiate the reporter's suspicions, the reporter (whether mandated to report or not) is protected from legal retaliation *if the report was made in "good faith"*. This protection from legal retaliation is called *immunity*. Without immunity, a reporter could potentially be held liable for defamation, infliction of emotional distress, and other offenses if the report is not substantiated.

The "good faith" immunity provisions were included in all states' laws to encourage the making of reports, even when the reporter is unsure that abuse or neglect has occurred (Kalichman, 1999). Making a report in good faith means that the reporter has reason to believe that the allegation made is true to the best of his or her knowledge. The reporter does not have to be sure that the allegations are true. In fact, reporters are not supposed to investigate suspicions before making a report. As long as the reporter has reason to believe that the child in question is being abused or neglected, a resulting report will be considered to be made in good faith.

In more than 15 states and the District of Columbia, there is a "presumption of good faith" for reports made by all persons, not just mandated reporters. This means that in these states, the burden is on the person accusing the reporter to prove that the report was not made in good faith. The reporter does not have to show evidence to prove that the report was made in good faith unless the accuser has convinced the court otherwise beyond a preponderance of the evidence. In that case, the reporter will then have the opportunity to rebut the case.

In a few states, including California, the mandated reporter benefits from absolute immunity. Absolute immunity means that immunity is provided to mandated reporters regardless of whether or not the report is made in good faith. In these states, however, absolute immunity is only provided to mandated reporters.

In all states, regardless of whether there is a legal "presumption" of good faith, the burden is on the person filing the claim against the reporter to prove that the report was *not* made in good faith. This is a difficult legal burden to meet.

Legal immunity does not mean that the mandated reporter cannot or will not be sued for making the report, although such lawsuits are very rare. However, mandated reporters should be able to successfully defend themselves by asserting immunity. In some states, such as California, there are provisions in which mandated reporters can be reimbursed for expenses made to defend themselves in such suits.

It is important to note that behaviors outside the reporting of the suspected child abuse or neglect are not protected through statutory immunity, even in absolute immunity states, such as California. For instance, if a mandated reporter not only shares the report with CPS but also broadcasts the allegations through social media and the allegations are found to be untrue, then the mandated reporter may be liable for damage to reputation caused by the social media postings but not liable for damage caused by the report to CPS.

What Are the Consequences for Not Fulfilling Your Legal Obligations as a Mandated Reporter?

The "flip-side" of protections for making reports in good faith, are laws that punish reporters who make reports in "bad faith". The law in almost all states provides civil and/or criminal liability for knowingly filing a false report. The reporter must have "willfully" or "intentionally" made a false report of child abuse or neglect. This means that the reporter knew that the report was false or knew that it was likely that the report was false. Cases of false reporting by mandated reporters are few and far between, although there are many cases of false reporting by non-mandated reporters. Disgruntled neighbors and ex-lovers have been found to file false reports in an effort to disrupt or injure a person or family. In states with absolute immunity for reporting by mandated reporters, there are no legal repercussions if a mandated reporter makes a false report, but a false report filed by a non-mandated reporter would still be subject to criminal or civil action.

Most states classify false reporting as a crime at the low level of a misdemeanor. In a handful of states, the offense of filing a false child abuse report is a higher-level crime—a felony. Criminal penalties include fines ranging from $100 to $5,000 or from 90 days to five years in jail or prison. In a few states, reporters who are found to have filed more than one false report are subject to even harsher penalties.

In addition to criminal consequences, reporters who make false reports can also be subject to civil liability for compensatory and/or punitive damages awarded by a court. Compensatory damages are meant to address any losses that were caused by the false report. The losses need not be financial, but the award will generally be monetary. Such compensatory damages can cover damage to reputation, disruption caused by the investigation, and even assault and battery for unwarranted physical examinations of children in response to a false report.

People who make false reports may also be forced to pay punitive damages. Punitive damages are meant to "punish" bad behavior. Punitive damages generally involve a large monetary award that is above and beyond the actual damages caused by the report.

False reporting is generally not a concern for mandated reporters, but failing to report when the law requires one is a perennial concern. Even though millions of reports of suspected child abuse and neglect are made every year in the United States, research has shown that there are many cases that are never reported (Delaronde et al., 2000). The law in all states is designed to encourage reports by providing immunity for reporters but also by punishing the failure to report suspected child abuse or neglect.

Penalties for failure to report child abuse or neglect only attach when it can be shown that the mandated reporter knew or should have known that he or she was legally obligated to report particular suspicions. This standard can be further classified as a "willful failure" of the mandated reporter to fulfill the legal duty to report suspected child abuse or neglect. Some mandated reporters may fail to make a report because they feel they do not have the time to make the report or be involved in an investigation. Other mandated reporters may fail to make a report because previous experiences with CPS were troubling, and they do not want to go through a similar experience. Willful failure can even include situations where the mandated reporter simply delays making the report.

The law is specifically designed to provide strong penalties for failing to make a report. In 48 states (not including Maryland or Wyoming), there are criminal penalties for mandated reporters who fail to make a report when required by law. In most states, failure to report is a misdemeanor. Misdemeanor offenses are usually punishable by fine, but in some states, misdemeanor offenses can carry a sentence of jail time or probation. In some states, failure to report serious allegations (such as physical and sexual abuse) carries stronger penalties, such as being classified a felony offense. In some states, when a reporter fails to report child abuse or neglect more than once, harsher criminal penalties can be expected. In states where there is not a specific provision for criminal liability for failure to report, such an offense may be considered a crime under general criminal law (Besharov, 1990).

In addition to criminal liability, a mandated reporter who fails to make a report when required by law may also be subject to civil liability. In a civil case, a mandated reporter who fails to make a report when required by law to do so can be held responsible to pay for damages to the child and/or the child's family incurred after the report should have been made (Besharov, 1990). For instance, the mandated reporter will not be held responsible for the damage of the abuse or neglect that occurred before the reporter should have made a report. However, the mandated reporter will be held responsible for any damage as a result of abuse or neglect that occurs *after* the reporter should have made a report.

Even if a given state does not have specific civil liability provisions for a mandated reporter's failure to report suspected child abuse or neglect, such failure may be considered negligence under general civil law. Negligence is a civil action most often used against professionals, such as social workers, who are bound by ethical responsibilities to protect others in addition to their legal responsibilities as mandated reporters. To be held liable for negligence, a mandated reporter must be shown to have a duty that he or she failed to fulfill. The failure to fulfill the duty must have caused damage. The mandated reporter would then be liable for any damage caused by failure to fulfill his or her duty.

One duty that may be implicated by a failure to report child abuse or neglect is the duty of mental health professionals to protect persons from likely harm, regardless of any duty to protect client confidentiality. This duty to protect was first determined by the California Supreme Court in the case of *Tarasoff v. Regents of the University of California* (1976). In this case, a psychologist, Dr. Lawrence Moore, was held responsible for failing to protect Tatiana Tarasoff from impending danger by one of Dr. Moore's clients. The client, Prosenjit Poddar, told Dr. Moore during a therapy session at the University of California Mental Health Clinic that he intended to kill Ms. Tarasoff because she rejected his romantic advances. Although Dr. Moore reported these statements to the campus police, and Mr. Poddar was briefly held in their custody, Dr. Moore neither contacted the local police department, nor warned Ms. Tarasoff herself. The court found fault in Dr. Moore for these failures and determined that it is the responsibility of mental health professionals to protect a potential victim from impending harm.

Although the *Tarasoff* duty was a result of case law in California, and therefore the court's holding was only applicable to California, subsequent changes to the statutory law as well as similar court cases in other states generally codified this duty across the country. Therefore, social workers generally have a legal duty to warn known potential victims of impending harm. The *Tarasoff* duty can be considered relevant to child abuse and neglect reporting in that a report to CPS is made to protect children from future harm.

Although research shows that mandated reporters fail to report almost half of their suspicions to CPS (Delaronde et al., 2000), mandated reporters are very rarely prosecuted for failure to report. Even though such cases are few and far between, they are often the focus of high-profile media coverage (Kalichman, 1999). A case involving teachers in New York State is representative of the national experience.

In Bedford Hills, New York, a northern suburb of New York City, school officials did not report suspicions of sexual abuse of a young female student, failed to protect a girl from further abuse, and threatened the jobs of teachers and administrators alike. In late 2005, the mother of an elementary school student made a report to a teacher in charge of the school that her daughter told her a 9-year-old classmate had sex with an adult (Saunders, 2007). The school responded by performing an internal investigation. The alleged victim's teachers were asked if they noticed anything wrong with the student that would suggest sexual abuse. When none of the student's teachers reported any behavior out of the ordinary, the school did not report the suspicions to CPS. When the mother of the alleged victim pursued criminal action against her paramour for raping her daughter, it became known that the school was aware of the allegations and had failed to report them to CPS. Criminal charges were filed against the principal. The charges were later dismissed after the principal agreed to share her story in a number of trainings to mandated reporters across New York State. Civil charges were also filed by the alleged victim's mother against the principal and involved teachers (Whitaker, 2006). The principal lost her position at the school. In response to the case, New York State increased its training efforts in the schools for mandated reporters.

It is important to note that the mother of the classmate also failed to make a report to CPS, but since New York State is not a Universal Mandated Reporting state, she was not a mandated reporter, so she could not be held liable. The case highlights an important point for mandated reporters to consider. They should not be asking themselves, "Can I prove child abuse occurred in this instance?" Instead, they should ask, "Does it make reasonable sense that I am suspicious that abuse might have occurred?" In this case, it was reasonable to believe that sexual abuse might have occurred merely by the fact that the child shared the information with her classmates, even if there were no behavioral indicators and even if she denied the abuse when asked.

As indicated by the Bedford Hills case, mandated reporters' employment may be in jeopardy if they fail to fulfill their duties as mandated reporters. Failing to fulfill their duties as mandated reporters can serve as "cause" for the termination of even the most secure job.

If a mandated reporter fails to report suspected child maltreatment, the individual's professional license may also be in jeopardy. In states where social workers are licensed professionals, the law generally requires them to follow all applicable federal, state, and local laws. Failure to report child abuse when mandated to do so would be a failure to follow state law. Therefore, social workers could be subject to state license board intervention in the form of fines, suspension, or even license revocation.

Professional associations, such as the NASW, may sanction (including expulsion from the professional organization), censure, or suggest corrective action for social workers who are found to have failed in the legal and ethical obligation to report suspected child abuse.

What Are the Criticisms and Concerns About Mandated Reporting?

Although it is clear that child maltreatment cases are increasingly reported and adjudicated at least partly due to mandated reporting, the system of mandated reporting continues to receive criticism. Some skeptics posit that mandating professionals to report child abuse is simply a waste of valuable resources. One argument is that *everyone* is morally obligated to make reports of suspected child abuse. By mandating that certain groups of people are required by law to report their suspicions, those who are not legally required to make reports will not do so, leaving many children vulnerable to further abuse and neglect. Underreporting, overreporting, and discrimination are three specific criticisms of the current mandated reporting system.

Research shows that more than half of mandated reporters fail to report cases where they suspect child abuse and maltreatment (Delaronde et al., 2000). Mandated reporters cite a variety of reasons for not reporting. They often lack certainty about what cases are reportable (Zellman & Antler, 1990). Most professionals understand that certain physical acts against a child are reportable, such as physical and sexual abuse (Alvarez et al., 2004). Neglect, however, is often cited as being complicated to identify and, therefore, it can be more difficult to determine when to report. However, neglect constitutes most of the reportable cases (Alvarez et al., 2004). Even less clear are cases of emotional abuse (Alvarez et al., 2004).

Mandated reporters also cite confusion or concerns about the process of reporting suspected child abuse or neglect (Kesner & Robinson, 2002; Reiniger et al., 1995). Some mandated reporters believe they have insufficient evidence to make a report (Delaronde et al., 2000). Others argue that reporting may produce more harm than good. Some mandated reporters suggest that the reporter can better handle the case than child protection services (Delaronde et al., 2000). Mandated reporters with a therapeutic relationship with the family cite ethical conflict as a deterrent to reporting (Delaronde et al., 2000). Mandated reporters have also expressed concerns with their internal agency procedures/protocols as to when a case may be reportable (Alvarez et al., 2004).

No matter what the reason for not reporting suspected maltreatment, it is clear that many children are left at risk because many mandated reporters do not report their suspicions, even though they are legally obligated to do so.

Underreporting is not the only problem with the current state of mandated reporting. Overreporting of suspicions is also an issue. More than half of all reports of child abuse and maltreatment are ultimately unsubstantiated (US DHHS, Administration on Children, Youth, and Families, 2007). As a result of overreporting, many children and families suffer from unwarranted intrusion and disruption. Additionally, overreporting puts added pressure on an already overburdened system by requiring unnecessary investigations.

Overreporting overwhelms services that are supposed to be targeted to at-risk children and families (Ainsworth, 2002; Besharov, 1986).

In most states, mandated reporters are not required to receive training on their responsibilities. As a result, mandated reporters may fulfill their legal obligation to report without understanding if their suspicions rise to a level that requires a report.

Beyond underreporting and overreporting, racially disproportionate reporting is another troubling issue. Children of color, including African-American, Hispanic, and Native American children, are reported at higher rates than in the general population. Disproportionate reporting may be due in part to disparate rates of poverty amongst non-white Americans, but bias may also contribute to this phenomenon. As a result, although intended to protect children and families, mandated reporting of child maltreatment may also contribute to institutional classism and racism.

Policymakers who designed the original mandated reporting legislation were concerned that, because poor and disenfranchised families are more likely to come in contact with mandated reporters than wealthier families, they might be more likely to be reported. Additionally, professionals who are mandated reporters may be less likely to report wealthier families, even when they have reasonable suspicion. The mandated reporter may feel that the wealthier family does not need to be involved in CPS. Instead, the mandated reporter may work with the family to improve their functioning without alerting CPS. Other mandated reporters may choose not to report wealthier families because they are concerned that they will lose potential clients if they report their suspicions. Efforts to prevent discrimination in the reporting and investigation of child abuse and maltreatment are needed. Improving training for mandated reporters is one way to address this concern.

Researchers and policymakers have consistently called for increased and improved, training for mandated reporters. Some states require training for some mandated reporters, but most are not trained. Some states require social workers to attend training once in a lifetime in order to receive their license. Some states may include mandated reporter training in their continuing education programs for licensed social workers. Social workers who work in the school system may be required by state law to complete training annually in some states. Other social workers who conduct custody evaluations for the courts may also be required to complete training, whether once or on a continuing basis.

How Can Social Workers Help Clients After a Report Has Been Made?

Social workers are unlike many other reporters of suspected child maltreatment. Oftentimes, the role of the social worker does not end after a report is made. They must continue to work with the client and/or CPS.

CPS often contacts the reporter during the investigation. CPS may also reach out to service providers for families who are the subject of reports of suspected child maltreatment, even if those providers *did not* make the report. When social workers communicate with CPS, regardless of circumstance, it is important to remember there are still ethical expectations for protecting confidential client communications. Even though the law allows you to breach client confidentiality in order to make a report of suspected child maltreatment to CPS, you are required to minimize the breach. Generally, reporters should limit the information shared with CPS to that which informed the decision to make the report and information received since making the report that is relevant to the concerns expressed in the report (Lau et al., 2008).

If the social worker did not make the report, and CPS is seeking information about a client, before providing any information the social worker should require CPS to secure a release from the client or a court-ordered subpoena. At all times, social workers should provide the minimal amount of confidential client information necessary to fulfill their legal and ethical obligations.

Negotiating a relationship with CPS after making a report may seem easy compared to figuring out how to work with a continuing client. Should the social worker tell the client s/he made the report, or not? The law *does not* require anyone to inform a client when a mandated report is made about the client or the client's family.

When making the decision whether to tell a client that a report was made to CPS, safety should be the primary consideration. If there are reasonable concerns that anyone's safety would be in jeopardy if a client was notified that a report was made to CPS, then the client should not be so informed.

If no one's safety is at risk, then a social worker can choose to tell the client about the report. The social worker should consider the impact that such a disclosure will have on the relationship with the client and on the client's participation in services he/she is receiving from the social worker. A client may decide that he/she no longer wants to receive services from a social worker who made a report to CPS. While this decision may seem unfortunate, you also need to remember that the client has the right to self-determination (National Association of Social Workers, 2008, 1.02). In the case where a client refuses to continue services with a social worker because a report was made to CPS, the social worker should provide the client the opportunity to work with someone else within the agency or a referral to a social worker in another setting.

If a social worker decides to *not inform* the client of a report to CPS, the social worker should still consider the impact that this omission might have on the professional relationship with the client. If a client knows a report was made to CPS but does not know who made it, the client may seek to process feelings with the social worker without knowing that they are talking to the individual responsible for the report.

Making the decision to report suspected child maltreatment is never easy, even for a seasoned professional. However, a thorough understanding of the process of reporting and an appreciation for the complexities of the obligation can allay some of the biggest concerns.

Case Scenarios and Questions

Case One

A school social worker made a report because she and a classroom teacher believed a child was being sexually abused. The investigation ended, and the report was not substantiated. The parents figured out that the school made the report and told the principal that they are going to sue the school.

1   What legal provisions protect the reporter from liability?

Case Two

A clinical social worker living in Brooklyn, New York, was traveling home from a music concert on the subway. The social worker witnessed a parent yell "shut up" at a young child who was babbling, and the parent called the non-verbal child "stupid". When the child did not remain quiet, the parent smacked the child across the face. A few bystanders on the train, including the social worker, confronted the parent about the behavior and told the parent to stop or they would call the police. The parent told them to "mind their own business" and got off the train at the next stop.

1   Was the social worker mandated to report the parent to child protective services?
2   What if the social worker was riding a commuter train in nearby New Jersey?

Resources

- In order to determine where to make a report of suspected child maltreatment in ANY state, consult the Child Welfare Gateway's listing of state-level hotlines: https://www.childwelfare.gov/topics/responding/reporting/how/
- If you need assistance in determining whether you need to make a report of suspected maltreatment, you can either call your state hotline for guidance or contact Childhelp. Childhelp is a national organization that provides crisis assistance and other counseling and referral services. The Childhelp National Child Abuse Hotline is staffed 24 hours a day, 7 days a week by professional crisis counselors who have access to a database of 55,000 emergency, social service, and support resources. All calls are anonymous. Contact them at 1.800.4.A.CHILD (1.800.422.4453).

References

Ainsworth, F. (2002). Mandatory Reporting of Child Abuse and Neglect: Does It Really Make a Difference? *Child & Family Social Work*, 7 (1), 57–63.

Alvarez, K.M., Kenny, M.C., Donohue, B., & Carpin, K.M. (2004). Why are Professionals Failing to Initiate Mandated Reports of Child Maltreatment, and Are There any Empirically Based Training Programs to Assist Professionals in the Reporting Process? *Aggression and Violent Behavior*, 9, 563–578.

Besharov, D.J. (1986). Unfounded Allegations: A New Child Abuse Problem. *Public Interest*, 83 (Spring), 18–33.

Besharov, D.J. (1990). *Recognizing Child Abuse: A Guide for the Concerned*. New York: The Free Press.

Child Abuse Prevention and Treatment Act. (1974). 42 U.S.C. § 51106a(b)(2)(A) (iv).

Delaronde, S., King, G., Bendel, R., & Reece, R. (2000). Opinions Among Mandated Reporters Toward Child Maltreatment Reporting Policies. *Child Abuse and Neglect*, 24 (7), 901–910.

Hutchison, E.D. (1993). Mandatory Reporting Laws: Child Protective Case Finding Gone Awry? *Social Work*, 38 (1), 56–63.

In Re Gault, 387 U.S. 1 (1967).

Kalichman, S.C. (1999). *Mandated Reporting of Suspected Child Abuse: Ethics, Law, and Policy*. Washington, DC: American Psychological Association.

Kempe, C.H., Silverman, F.N., Steele, B.F., Droegemueller, W., & Silver, H.K. (1962). The Battered-Child Syndrome. *Journal of the American Medical Association*, 181 (1), 17–24.

Kesner, J.E. & Robinson, M. (2002). Teachers and Mandated Reporters of Child Maltreatment: Comparison with Legal, Medical, and Social Services Reporters. *Children & Schools*, 24 (4), 222–231.

Lau, K.J., Krase, K.S., & Morse, R. (2008). *Mandated Reporting of Child Abuse and Neglect: A Practical Guide for Social Workers*. New York: Springer.

National Association of Social Workers. (2008). *Code of Ethics of the National Association of Social Workers*. Washington, DC: National Association of Social Workers.

Reiniger, A., Robison, E., & McHugh, M. (1995). Mandated Training of Professionals: A Means for Improving Reporting of Suspected Child Abuse. *Child Abuse and Neglect*, 19 (1), 63–69.

Saunders, S. (2007). What You Need to Know About Child Abuse: A Cautionary Tale from Bedford Hills. *New York Teacher*. Latham, NY: NYSUT.

Sussman, A. & Cohen, S. (1975). *Reporting Child Abuse and Neglect: Guidelines for Legislation*. Cambridge, MA: Ballinger Publishing Company.

Tarasoff v. Regents of the University of California, 17 Cal. 3d 425 (1976).

US DHHS, Administration on Children, Youth, and Families. (2007). *Child Maltreatment 2005*. Washington, DC: US Government Printing Office.

US DHHS, Administration on Children, Youth, and Families. (2015). *Child Maltreatment 2005*. Washington, DC: US Government Printing Office.

Whitaker, B. (2006). Bedford Hills Principal Will Have Charge Dropped. *New York Times*, December 10, p. 2.

Zellman, G.L. & Antler, S. (1990). Mandated Reporters and CPS: A Study in Frustration. *Public Welfare*, 48 (1), 30–37.

12 Prevention and Preservation

Thinking about Prevention

Picture, for a minute, an alternate universe, but one very much like our own:

A family with a school-aged child was travelling along a quiet road. They came upon a small village with an unexpected amount of activity in the center of town. The family parked their car and got out to see what was happening. They realized there was commotion on the banks of the river that runs through the town. As they approached the river, they saw the townspeople removing dozens of floating baskets from the water. The family realized that the baskets held babies and young children. The visitors asked a townsperson, "What is going on here?" The townsperson responded, "We are saving the babies. They keep floating down the river. There are so many of them, but we are a small town. We can't save them all before they get past our town. Can you help?"

The parents looked at each and nodded, "Of course we can!" As they readied themselves for the task at hand, they looked for their child, who was walking away from them with a purpose. "Where are you going?" the parents asked "The town and the children need our help," they said to the child.

"The town and the children DO need our help," the child answered. "That's why I'm going upriver to stop whomever is putting these baskets INTO the river."

(Adapted from Guggenheim, 2005)

This story illustrates a common theme in social services in the United States and around the world. When a problem presents itself, it is often easiest to respond by minimizing the outcome. However, in many cases, the problem itself could be prevented from happening in the first place.

What Are the Different Levels of Prevention?

We all know that the word "prevention" relates to stopping a phenomenon from occurring. So, when we talk about prevention in the context of child maltreatment, we are talking about efforts to stop children from being maltreated.

When we talk about prevention as a child maltreatment intervention, it is important to note that there are different levels: primary, secondary, and tertiary.

Primary Prevention

Primary prevention relates to efforts aimed at the general population that seek to reduce or stop child maltreatment from occurring (Children's Bureau, 2018). Primary prevention programs are universal in nature, meaning that they serve the population, children, and families, regardless of status, risk, or precondition. For instance, primary prevention programs for child maltreatment include school-based psycho-educational programs to increase awareness of child sexual abuse, public service messages on television and radio about positive parenting, as well as newspaper and media campaigns about shaken baby syndrome.

Primary prevention efforts are often criticized for being too vague and not targeting those most in need. It is also hard to use research to support the efficacy of primary prevention efforts since they are broad, and the impacts are harder to calculate statistically.

Secondary Prevention

Secondary prevention relates to efforts targeted at segments of the population at higher risk for child maltreatment. For instance, research consistently shows that children living in poverty are more likely to be victims of child maltreatment. Therefore, an example of a secondary prevention program would be one that offers parenting support services to low-income families in an effort to prevent child maltreatment. Research also finds that children with special needs are at increased risk of child maltreatment. Therefore, a program designed to provide parents of special needs children with respite services could be considered a secondary prevention program.

Secondary prevention efforts are often well received since they target and support groups that are at-risk. Secondary prevention efforts often have supportive research since it is easy to compare outcomes for those who received the targeted services with outcomes for those at risk of child maltreatment who did not receive the services.

Tertiary Prevention

Tertiary (i.e., third-level) prevention efforts relate to services provided to children and families where child maltreatment has occurred in an effort to prevent additional maltreatment from occurring and to reduce the negative consequences of past maltreatment. Tertiary prevention programs may include substitute care for impacted children, individual or family therapy, treatment programs for parental addictions, and parenting support groups.

Intensive Family Preservation Services (IFPS) is a form of tertiary prevention often used for families identified as being at high risk for continued child maltreatment. "Preservation" speaks to the long-standing policy goal of keeping a family together or reunifying a family that has been separated through the use of substitute care. Family preservation services, therefore, relate to efforts designed to advance the goal of family preservation.

How Has Policy Impacted Prevention and Preservation Efforts?

If you remember the chapters on the history of the child welfare system, you will have noted that the system developed as a response to child maltreatment that was already occurring. Therefore, the system evolved largely as a tertiary prevention model, responding to acts of identified maltreatment. However, the form of tertiary prevention most often utilized by early private organizations was substitute care.

In the early child welfare system, actors were primarily private organizations funded completely through donations from rich philanthropists. Funders placed an emphasis on "saving" children from "bad" families. During the early period there were community-based social work services, such as settlement houses and charity organization societies, that can be considered forms of primary and secondary prevention organizations. They focused on child welfare services, in particular, and expended most of their efforts removing children from their homes.

As local, state, and federal governments became increasingly involved in the provision of child welfare services in the mid-to-late twentieth century, primary and secondary prevention efforts gained traction, particularly as a way to reduce the need for exorbitant financial expenditures associated with the use of substitute care. With the passage of CAPTA in 1974, the federal government began to reimburse states for many of the costs associated with substitute care. In the next five years, the number of children in foster care skyrocketed, and the cost to the federal budget increased proportionally.

In response, the AACWA of 1980 was designed and passed into law. It required states to expend "reasonable efforts" to keep families together before placing a child in foster care. Preservation efforts were designed to help states meet the federal mandate. Today, almost 40 years later, "reasonable efforts" are still required, and policymakers have developed additional requirements to encourage the child welfare system to preserve families whenever possible.

The combination of federal policy and state and local practices has increased prevention and preservation efforts. In February 2018, the Family First Prevention Services Act was passed into federal law. The Act includes long-overdue reforms of the child welfare system aimed to keep children safely in their homes whenever possible. When it is determined that substitute care is necessary, the law emphasizes placement in the most family-like setting appropriate to the child's needs (Children's Defense Fund, 2018).

Evidence-Based Practice in Prevention and Preservation

Similar to every other area of social work practice, there is important emphasis on evidence-base practices in both the prevention of child maltreatment and family preservation. Evidence of program efficacy is particularly important because the major sources of funding, the federal and state governments, are under constant scrutiny and must justify every tax dollar spent. As a result, programs that aim to prevent child maltreatment or preserve families in their homes must be able to support their existence with research to ensure they are classified as "evidence-based". The following are examples of two evidence-based programs that have been adopted in multiple jurisdictions, in part because their efficacy has been demonstrated through research.

Family Connections (FC)

Family Connections (FC) is a "multi-faceted, community-based service program that works with vulnerable families in their homes and in the context of their neighborhoods to help them meet the basic needs of their children and prevent child maltreatment" (DePanfilis et al., 2009). The FC program was designed by faculty of the University of Maryland School of Social Work.

The FC program is a secondary prevention program that involves four core components:

1 emergency assistance (or crisis intervention services),
2 home-visiting family intervention, including family assessments, outcome-driven service plans, and individual and family counseling,
3 a family center model of practice, and
4 multi-family supportive and recreational activities that, organically, provide families with a social/community support structure.

The FC program developers secured funding for a Baltimore-based pilot from the Department of Health and Human Services, Office of Child Abuse and Neglect. In the initial program, randomly-selected families that met risk inclusion criteria but were not currently involved with CPS received FC services for three or nine months. The initial experimental study found that families and children receiving FC services showed positive improvements in family protective factors, diminished risk factors, and improved child safety and behaviors. Additionally, families that received the services for a longer period of time had higher levels of improvement and fewer risk factors.

As a result, additional funding was secured so that the FC program could be replicated at eight sites across the country. Each replication site had a unique focus on a different population or risk factor. For instance, the Los Angeles replication of the FC program focused on serving families from the Asian-Pacific Islander community. In Detroit the program focused efforts on serving black families. The Tennessee replication focused on low-income families in a rural area. Evaluations of these replication sites have been positive and encouraged further replication to additional sites.

Homebuilders®

Homebuilders® is an evidence-based program designed to provide services to families with children at imminent risk of placement into substitute care. Homebuilders® is the oldest and best-documented Intensive Family Pre-servation Services (IFPS) program in the United States (Institute for Family Development, 2018).

Homebuilders® provides intensive, in-home crisis intervention, counseling, and life-skills education. The program's goal is to prevent unnecessary out-of-home placements of children. The program serves families involved in the child protection and juvenile justice systems. Since children with mental health disorders are at an increased risk for involvement in the child protection and juvenile justice systems, Homebuilders® also works within the children's mental health system to broaden the continuum of care and reduce overreliance on residential treatment and psychiatric hospitalization.

The structure of Homebuilders® involves three to five two-hour in-person/home sessions per week, with additional contact via telephone. On average, the program lasts for four to six weeks, followed by additional follow-up visits over the subsequent three to four months.

Homebuilders® has been the subject of extensive programmatic assessment since 1974. Over 40 years of research has consistently shown the program's efficacy, earning it a California Evidence-Based Clearinghouse for Child Welfare (2018) rating of "2" for being "supported by research evidence". As a result of its proven efficacy, Homebuilders® has been replicated by at least six different states.

Case Scenarios and Questions

Case One

David was born eight weeks premature and weighed only five pounds at birth. His father died four weeks before he was born in a work accident on a construction site. His mother seems disinterested in David at the hospital.

1   What prevention intervention(s) is/are appropriate?
2   What level(s) of prevention is/are appropriate?

Case Two

Joanne is a single mother of three young children. She is a survivor of intimate partner violence and is in recovery for opiate addiction. Her children were removed from her care when she was actively using drugs. She has been clean and compliant for ten months and is in an in-patient treatment program that allows her children to stay with her.

1   What prevention intervention(s) is/are appropriate?
2   What level(s) of prevention is/are appropriate?

Case Three

Rural farming communities across the country are experiencing an opiate addiction crisis of epic proportions. #FarmTownStrong is a responsive campaign funded by two private, non-profit organizations—the American Farm Bureau Federation and the National Farmers Union—to increase awareness of addiction and opportunities for prevention and treatment.

1   While not intentionally designed to prevent child maltreatment, what level of prevention does this initiative fit the definition of?

Questions

1   What policies can you recommend our society adopt for primary prevention of child maltreatment?
2   What factors impact the likelihood of your recommendations being adopted and implemented?

References

California Evidence-Based Clearinghouse for Child Welfare. (2018). Homebuilders®. *CEBC: The California Evidence-Based Clearinghouse for Child Welfare.* Retrieved from: http://www.cebc4cw.org/program/homebuilders/detailed.

Children's Bureau. (2018). Framework for prevention of child maltreatment. *Child Welfare Information Gateway.* Retrieved from: https://www.childwelfare.gov/top ics/preventing/overview/framework.

Children's Defense Fund. (2018). The Family First Prevention Services Act: Historic Reforms to the Child Welfare System Will Improve Outcomes for Vulnerable Children. *Children's Defense Fund.* Retrieved from: https://www.childrensdefense. org/wp-content/uploads/2018/08/family-first-detailed-summary.pdf.

DePanfilis, D., Filene, J.H., & Brodowski, M.L. (2009). Introduction to Family Connections and the National Replication Effort. *Protecting Children,* 24 (3), 4–13.

Guggenheim, M. (2005). *What's Wrong with Children's Rights?* Cambridge, MA: Harvard University Press.

Institute for Family Development. (2018). Homebuilders®. *Institute for Family Development.* Retrieved from: http://www.institutefamily.org/programs_ifps.asp.

13 Substitute Care

Types of Substitute Care

Shelter Care

Shelter care is typically used as a temporary first placement for children coming into the child welfare system. Shelter care is meant to house children until a "permanent" home can be found, such as kinship placement or foster care. Unfortunately, because of the shortage of foster homes, especially for adolescents, many children end up staying in shelter care for long periods of time until they can reunite with parents. A study of shelter care by Leon, Bai, Fuller, and Busching (2016) found that older children with no option for kinship placement were more likely to be placed and stay in shelter care for longer periods of time. Specifically, shelter stays tend to be longer for children 12 to 17 years of age, children who are a racial minority, and children who have mental or physical challenges (Oakes & Freundlich, 2005). Additionally, children who enter shelter care as a first placement tend to have disrupted placements during their time in the child welfare system (Wulczyn et al., 2007). Shelter care is also more expensive than traditional foster care (DeSena et al., 2005). Some of the negative aspects of shelter care include overcrowding, abuse, exposure to violence (*B.H. v. McDonald*, 1988; *Ward v. Kearney*, 2000), and, as mentioned above, long stays lasting six months or more (*Brian A. v. Sundquist*, 2001).

Kinship Care

Kinship or fictive kin care involves relatives or close family friends caring for children who need out-of-home placement. Kinship care providers can be grandparents, aunts, uncles, cousins, and sometimes family friends or neighbors. In some states, kinship providers are required to attend the same training as foster parents. Some states require them to have their homes licensed, especially if they receive a stipend to care for the child. Kinship care is the first type of out-of-home placement considered for all children because it can decrease the additional trauma of being removed from the home. In 2018,

32% of children in foster care were placed in relatives' homes (AFCARS Report, 2019).

Foster Care

Foster care placement occurs for children when they cannot stay at home and they do not have a relative (kinship care) to care for them. In 2018, 46% of children in foster care were placed in non-relative homes (AFCARS Report, 2019). In order to become a foster parent, most states require training, home-study, and licensure that includes a home inspection. Foster homes are licensed for a specific number of children, including the foster parent's children. Generally, the rules require a foster home to have a bed for each child, and the foster parent's income must be sufficient to support the family as well as any foster children placed in the home. Foster parents receive monthly stipends; however, the stipend is a small amount of money intended to cover the costs of food, clothing, and other needs of the child. It is not considered a payment to the foster parent. Therapeutic foster care is more intensive care for children with behavioral or emotional issues. Therapeutic foster parents receive special training, and they are sometimes paid for caring for children with special needs. These homes have strict guidelines for the care of children, including restrictions on the accessibility of other children.

Some foster parents complete the process to become foster parents in order to foster-to-adopt children in the child welfare system. Sometimes, children placed in foster care are adopted by foster parents if the child cannot be reunited with biological parents. It may occur when the biological parents cannot complete the tasks in a case plan or provide a safe home free from abuse or neglect. A judge determines whether to terminate parental rights, freeing the child for adoption. Fostering to adopt is tricky. Federal law indicates that children should not be in any type of out-of-home placement longer than 24 months. With this in mind, child welfare workers and other child welfare team members have the goal of reuniting the child with the parents. This can be a challenge for foster parents who want to adopt. As part of the child welfare team, they must support and assist in the reunification process, even though they may have a desire to adopt the child in their care.

In the fall of 2018, it was estimated that about 437,283 children were in foster care in the United States (AFCARS Report, 2019). Half of the children who left foster care in 2018 reunited with primary caretakers and close to half left foster care after one year (AFCARS Report, 2019). There are negative factors associated with foster care. Foster care entry rates and the length of time children spend in foster care vary from state to state. Russell and Macgill (2015) stated that there is no way to balance removing a child from the home and the trauma they experience staying in foster care for long periods of time. The length of stay in foster care has been associated with certain child and parent characteristics. Children tend to have longer stays in foster care if they are younger, have special needs (CDC, 2012), or are African American (Summers et al., 2013). Family characteristics associated with longer foster care stays include parental incarceration; low socioeconomic status; having more than four children; social isolation; family disorganization, dissolution, and violence; parenting stress; poor parent-child relationships; and negative interpersonal interactions (CDC, 2012; Krug et. al., 2002; Sedlak et al., 2010). A study by Russell and Macgill (2015) identified community values, demographics, poverty, expenditure levels, policies on older youths, and performance measures as variables that predicted more lengthy stays in foster care.

Residential Services

Residential Treatment Center (RTC) placement is the most intensive and costly type of out-of-home care (Helgerson et al., 2007; Lyons, 2004). RTCs are used for youths who have severe emotional or behavioral problems and sometimes as a last resort because other placements have failed (Epstein, 2004; Foltz, 2004; McCurdy & McIntyre, 2004; Pfeiffer & Strzelecki, 1990). RTCs provide diagnostic services, intense therapeutic services, rehabilitative or secure treatment for delinquents, and services for children with severe special needs. Placement in an RTC can often lead to poor outcomes for youths, such as longer stays in care, unaddressed clinical concerns, and unplanned discharges (Foltz, 2004; Sunseri, 2005). Some of the problems associated with RTCs are staff issues, abuse of children during placement, and problems within the youth community, such as negative peer influence, violence, or child-on-child sexual abuse. In 2018, 6% of children were placed in institutions and 4% of children in foster care were placed in group homes (AFCARS Report, 2019). (See Figure 13.1 for the flowchart of steps followed for placement in substitute care.)

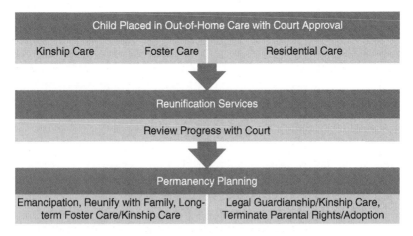

Figure 13.1 Steps Followed Through the Foster Care System for Placement in Substitute Care

Steps Followed Through the Foster Care System for Placement in Substitute Care

Team Decision-Making

Team decision-making is a relatively new concept in child welfare. The team decision-making process uses teams to inform and facilitate decision-making in child welfare cases. Teams typically consist of the parent, child, natural helpers, relatives, and professionals involved in case. Research indicates that when the team approach is used and parents are involved in case planning, case outcomes are more successful. Team decision-making has a number of benefits, such as team members bring a variety of perspectives to the case, parents are able to make choices and give input on their case, parents have a better understanding of the situation, and interventions are individualized. In addition, the team decision-making approach lightens the social worker's caseload, offers support and connections for the family, and promotes information sharing, transparency, and realistic casework.

Concurrent Case Planning

In addition to utilizing the team decision-making process, many child welfare agencies engage in concurrent case planning. In concurrent case planning, the child welfare worker prepares two different plans for the child that are implemented simultaneously. Concurrent case planning started in the early 1980s with the goal of providing a stable environment for a child, which promotes positive growth and development. The approach is influenced by the federal law that requires children be placed into a permanent home environment within 24 months of out-of-home placement (Goldman et al., 2003). Concurrent planning was developed as a structured approach to meet federal guidelines and ensure children move quickly through the child welfare system into a stable, safe, and permanent home (Goldman et al., 2003). The first plan focuses on the goal of reunification. The second, concurrent plan (back-up plan) focuses on another permanent home situation, such as guardianship, long-term kinship care, adoption, or independent living. The child and parent are fully informed of the concurrent plans.

Preparation for Leaving Foster Care

Jones (2014) indicates that foster youths need early preparation and skills for independent living, such as meal preparation, laundry, managing money, and self-care. In addition, they need study skills, positive work habits, transportation, and after-care services. A study by Jones (2014) indicated that after-care services could provide the support youths need and help them from feeling abandoned. After-care services would also entitle youths to case management, crisis intervention, mentoring, health insurance, and financial assistance (Jones, 2014).

Emancipation or Aging Out of Foster Care

While considerations for youths aging out of foster care is covered in more depth in Chapter 15, aging out and emancipation are important considerations in the discussion of substitute care.

Transition from foster care to independence is very difficult with little to no support. Many foster youths are unsuccessful and end up in poverty or homeless. Only 39–69% of children aging out of the system have earned a high school diploma (Barth et al., 2004; Courtney & Dworsky, 2005; Percora et al., 2005). Only 30% of former foster youth have attended at least one year of college (Courtney et al., 2007). Foster youth often leave foster care unemployed. When they do have a job, it is low or minimum wage (Berzin, 2008; Dworsky, 2005). Foster youth have high rates of using public assistance and living in poverty (Berzin, 2008; Curry & Abrams, 2015). Berzin (2008) found that poverty and low educational attainment were the two leading factors that hindered successful transition from foster care. Thirty to forty percent of previous foster youth have difficulty accessing health care (Courtney & Dworsky, 2005), and about the same percentage do not have health insurance (Pecora et al., 2005; Courtney & Dworsky, 2005). This is a concern because research shows that maltreatment in childhood increases the risk of health problems (SAMHSA, 2017), and many children in foster care have diagnosed mental health issues that go untreated after they age out (Landsverk et al., 2006). In addition, former foster youth also have higher rates of arrest and incarceration (Courtney & Dworsky, 2005).

Children can be successful after aging out of the foster care system. Graham, Schellinger, and Vaughn (2015) indicate that individual support and personal development are two important factors for successful aging out of the foster care system. Positive interpersonal relationships have been shown to increase academic success and decrease rates of homelessness for foster youth (Collins et al., 2010; Hass & Graydon, 2009; Klein, 2012; Pecora, 2012). Additionally, certain characteristics of an individual's "personal development" can be factors that contribute to successful aging out, such as self-esteem, perseverance, resilience, patience, focus, and emotional maturity (Graham et al., 2015; Osgood et al., 2010; Scales & Leffert, 2004; Search Institute, 2014).

References

Barbell, K. & Freundlich, M. (2001). *Foster Care Today*. Washington, DC: Casey Family Programs.

Barth, R.P., Courtney, M., Berrick, J.D., & Albert, V. (2004). *From Child Abuse to Foster Care*. New York: Aldine de Gruyter.

Berzin, S.C. (2008). Difficulties in the Transition to Adulthood: Using Propensity Scoring to Understand What Makes Foster Youth Vulnerable. *Social Services Review*, 82 (2), 171–196.

B.H. v. McDonald, No. 88–C–5599 (1988).

Brian A. v. Sundquist, No. 3–00–0445 (2001).

CDC (Centers for Disease Control). (2012). Child Maltreatment: Risk and Protective Factors. *CDC: Centers for Disease Control and Prevention*. Retrieved from: http://www.cdc.gov/violenceprevention/childmaltreatment/riskprotectivefactors.html.

Collins, M.E., Spencer, R., & Ward, R. (2010). Supporting Youth in Transition from Foster Care: Formal and Informal Connections. *Child Welfare*, 89 (1), 125–143.

Courtney, M. & Dworsky, A. (2005). *Midwest Evaluation of the Adult Functioning of Former Foster Youth: Outcomes at Age 19*. Chicago, IL: Chapin Hall Center for Children.

Courtney, M., Dworsky, A., Cusick, G., Havlicek, J., Perez, A., & Keller, T. (2007). *Midwest Evaluation of the Adult Functioning of Former Foster Youth: Outcomes at Age 21*. Chicago, IL: Chapin Hall Center for Children.

Curry, S.R. & Abrams, L.S. (2015). Housing and Social Support for Youth Aging Out of Foster Care: State of the Research Literature and Directions for Future Inquiry. *Child and Adolescent Social Work Journal*, 32, 143–153.

DeSena, A.D., Murphy, R.A., Douglas-Palumberi, H., Blau, G., Kelly, B., Horwitz, S.M., & Kaufman, J. (2005). SAFE Homes: Is it Worth the Cost?: An Evaluation of a Group Home Permanency Planning Program for Children Who First Enter Out-of-Home Care. *Child Abuse & Neglect*, 29, 627–643.

Dworsky, A. (2005). The Economic Self-Sufficiency of Wisconsin's Former Foster Youth. *Children and Youth Services Review*, 27 (10), 1085–1118.

Epstein, R.A., Jr. (2004). Inpatient and Residential Treatment Effects for Children and Adolescents: A Review and Critique. *Child and Adolescent Psychiatric Clinics of North America*, 13 (2), 411–428.

Foltz, R. (2004). The Efficacy of Residential Treatment: An Overview of the Evidence. *Residential Treatment for Children & Youth*, 22 (2), 1–19.

Goldman, J., Salus, M.K., Wolkott, D., & Kennedy, K.Y. (2003). *A Coordinated Response to Child Abuse and Neglect: The Foundation for Practice*. Washington, DC: US Department of Health and Human Services, Administration for Children and Families, Administration on Children, Youth, and Families, Children's Bureau, Office on Child Abuse and Neglect.

Graham, K.E., Schellinger, A.R., & Vaughn, L.M. (2015). Developing Strategies for Positive Change: Transitioning Foster Youth to Adulthood. *Children and Youth Services Review*, 54, 71–79.

Hass, M. & Graydon, K. (2009). Sources of Resiliency Among Successful Foster Youth. *Children and Youth Services Review*, 31, 457–463.

Helgerson, J., Martinovich, Z., Durkin, E., & Lyons, J.S. (2007). Differences in Outcome Trajectories of Children in Residential Treatment. *Residential Treatment for Children & Youth*, 22 (4), 67–79.

Jones, L.P. (2014). Former Foster Youth's Perspectives on Independent Living Preparation Six Months After Discharge. *Child Welfare*, 93 (1), 99–126.

Klein, R.A. (2012). Self-Concept Development Among Youth Participating in Transitional Living Program After Emancipation from Foster Care. Retrieved from ProQuest Digital Dissertations (AAT 3569390).

Krug, E.G., Dahlberg, L.L., Mercy, J.A., Zwi, A.B., & Lozano, R. (2002). *World Report on Violence and Health*. Geneva, Switzerland: World Health Organization.

Landsverk, J., Burns, B., Strambraugh, L., & Reutz, A. (2006). *Mental Health Care for Children and Adolescents in Foster Care: Review of Research Literature*. Seattle, WA: Casey Family Programs.

Leon, S.C., Bai, G.J., Fuller, A.K., & Busching, M. (2016). Emergency Shelter Utilization in Child Welfare: Who Goes to Shelter Care? How Long Do They Stay? *American Journal of Orthopsychiatry*, 86 (1), 49–60.

Lyons, J.S. (2004). *Redressing the Emperor: Improving our Children's Public Mental Health System*. Westport, CT: Praeger.

McCurdy, B.L. & McIntyre, E.K. (2004). "And what about residential...?": Re-Conceptualizing Residential Treatment as a Stop-Gap Service for Youth with Emotional and Behavioral Disorders. *Behavioral Interventions*, 19 (3), 137–158.

Oakes J.E. & Freundlich, M. (2005). *The Role of Emergency Care as a Child Welfare Service*. New York: Children's Rights.

Osgood, D.W., Foster, E.M., & Courtney, M.E. (2010). Vulnerable Populations and the Transition to Adulthood. *The Future of Children*, 20 (1), 209–229.

Pecora, P.J. (2012). Maximizing Educational Achievement of Youth in Foster Care and Alumni: Factors Associated with Success. *Children and Youth Services Review*, 34, 1121–1129.

Percora, P., Kessler, R., Williams, J., O'Brien, K., Downs, C., English, D., White, J., Hiripi, E., Wiggins, T., & Holmes, K. (2005). *Improving Family Foster Care: Findings from the Northwest Foster Care Alumni Studies*. Seattle, WA: Casey Family Programs.

Pfeiffer, S.I. & Strzelecki, S.C. (1990). Inpatient Psychiatric Treatment of Children and Adolescents: A Review of Outcome Studies. *Journal of the American Academy of Child and Adolescent Psychiatry*, 29 (6), 847–853.

Russell, J. & Macgill, S. (2015). Demographics, Policy, and Foster Care Rates: A Predictive Analytic Approach. *Children and Youth Services Review*, 58, 118–126.

SAMHSA (Substance Abuse and Mental Health Services Administration). (2017). Adverse Childhood Experiences. *Substance Abuse and Mental Health Services Administration*. Retrieved from: https://www.samhsa.gov/capt/practicing-effecti ve-prevention/prevention-behavioral-health/adverse-childhood-experiences.

Scales, P.C. & Leffert, N. (2004). *Developmental Assets: A Synthesis of the Scientific Research on Adolescent Development*. Minneapolis, MN: Search Institute.

Search Institute. (2014). Developmental Assets. *Search Institute*. Retrieved September 2014 from: http:// www.search-institute.org/research/developmental-assets.

Sedlak, A.J., Mettenburg, J., Basena, M., Peta, I., McPherson, K., & Greene, A. (2010). *Fourth National Incidence Study of Child Abuse and Neglect (NIS-4)*. Washington, DC: US Department of Health and Human Services. Retrieved from: http://www.law.harvard.edu/programs/about/cap/cap-conferences/rd-con ference/rd-conference-papers/sedlaknis.pdf.

Summers, A., Wood, S., & Russell, J. (2013). *Disproportionality Rates for Children of Color in Foster Care (Technical Assistance Bulletin)*. Reno, NV: National Council of Juvenile and Family Court Judges.

Sunseri, P.A. (2005). Children Referred to Residential Care: Reducing Multiple Placements, Managing Costs and Improving Treatment Outcomes. *Residential Treatment for Children & Youth,* 22 (3), 55–66.

The AFCARS Report: Preliminary FY 2018 Estimates as of August 22, 2019 (26) (U.S. Department of Health and Human Services [HHS], 2019), available at https:// www.acf.hhs.gov/cb/resource/afcars-report-26.

Ward v. Kearney, No. 98–7137 (2000).

Wulczyn, F.H., Chen, I., & Hilsop, K. (2007). *Foster Care Dynamics 2000–2005: A Report from the Multistate Foster Care Data Archive*. Chicago, IL: University of Chicago, Chapin Hall Center for Children.

14 Adoption

Adoption Simplified

While the current accepted purpose of adoption is to provide a safe and permanent home for a child whose birth parents cannot provide one, adoption is more simply defined as the legal process through which a child is assigned a parent other than the parent(s) the child had at birth. The practice of adoption developed across many different cultures and for various reasons. However, adoption, no matter the intent, is a legal process through which the rights and responsibilities of a parent are transferred to another person. It is important to note that in many cultures, families find no need for formal adoption. Informal arrangements for transfers of parental rights and responsibilities happen often and without court or government involvement. This chapter focuses primarily on formal adoption processes and less on informal arrangements.

History of Adoption

Adoption today is focused on providing the best possible life for a child. Adoption was developed, however, for a much different purpose. As outlined in Chapter 1, it was not until modern times that children's welfare became a major societal consideration. Therefore, it should come as no surprise that adoption was not originally designed to serve the needs of children.

Adoption was designed in ancient Greek and Roman societies to ensure the hereditary rights of powerful families. If a wealthy man had no male child (or no male child he deemed worthy), he could adopt an adult as his child and pass on to that individual his property and related rights. In ancient Indian and Chinese cultures, the adoption of adult men guaranteed rich and powerful men, who lacked the appropriate male heirs, access to spiritual and religious rites and protections after they died.

In fact, there was little practice of or need for the adoption of children in ancient times. Abandoned or orphaned children could more easily be claimed as slaves and servants. However, there were ancient cultures where orphaned or abandoned children of relatives would be adopted by kin, although these practices were rarely formalized through legal means.

As we learned in Chapter 1, formal adoption remained rare in the early history of the United States. Orphaned or abandoned children were instead placed in poorhouses or almshouses along with alcoholic and mentally ill adults. Eventually, orphanages were designed to serve the child population. However, orphanages were not designed as an intermediary step to child adoption. Instead they were a housing alternative for children until they became independent, working adults. It was not until the societal transformations of the mid-nineteenth century that child adoption became more prevalent and formalized in the United States.

In the mid-nineteenth century, Massachusetts, Mississippi, and Texas passed laws formalizing the adoption process for children. The laws in Mississippi and Texas, which were rooted in English Common Law derived from Greek and Roman theories, emphasized the transfer of real property, otherwise known as real estate, through adoption. The new law in Massachusetts, however, was the first to focus on the needs of the child. Massachusetts required a finding that the adoptive parents were "fit and proper". The law also had additional requirements, such as written consent from the biological parents, there had to be both an adoptive mother *and* an adoptive father, and the relationship between the child and the biological parents was completely severed. These four tenets largely remain in modern adoption law across the United States.

The Orphan Train movement of the mid-to-late nineteenth century, explained in further detail in Chapter 1, was the earliest practice focused on adoption of children in the United States. While the movement professed to serve the needs of children, the system was popular across the country because it met the needs of adoptive parents. Younger children were not the most desirable children in the program, which focused on Midwest farming communities. Instead, teenage boys who could serve as unpaid field and farm hands were amongst the most wanted.

The first White House Conference on the Child in 1910 marked a new era in child welfare. The focus was on meeting the unique needs of children and creating a system of checks and balances to ensure their well-being. With this change came a preference for foster care and adoption over institutionalizing children in orphanages. In recognition of the growing demand for child adoption, all states passed statutes to govern the process by 1929. The new processes were neither formulaic nor intended to preserve the transfer of property through hereditary rights. Instead, they were designed to ensure child safety and often involved some level of investigation of adoptive families before finalization.

Changing demographic patterns throughout the twentieth century further impacted the adoption landscape in the United States. Rapidly improving infant mortality rates meant more healthy children were being born and surviving in the US (CDC, 1999). The maternal mortality rate did not see similar improvements until almost 1950 (CDC, 1999). The combination of infant survival, maternal mortality, economic pressures from the Great Depression, and growing societal acceptance of adoption produced a rapid increase in the number of infants available for adoption in the United States.

The demand for adoption was not universal. By the 1950s, the demand for healthy, white infants by white couples outweighed their availability. Adoption of non-white babies was often limited by policy or practice to non-white couples. Healthy black and mixed-race infants were often available, but there was a missing synergy with non-white couples seeking to adopt. As a result, many healthy black and mixed-race infants were left in substitute care.

As contraception and abortion became more widely available in the 1960s and 1970s, and the stigma against single parenthood decreased, the number of healthy white babies available for adoption declined. The demand, however, did not. As a result, states and private agencies revisited their policies and practices. Interracial adoptions, adoptions of toddlers and older children, and adoptions of children with special needs became more prevalent. The demand generated by white couples seeking healthy white infants created a market for private adoption services and international adoptions.

The increase in interracial adoptions in the 1960s and 1970s, which coincided with the Civil Rights Movement, prompted significant backlash from professional and cultural groups. In 1968, the National Association of Black Social Workers (NABSW) Harambee was formed in San Francisco, California. Their original position statement clearly articulates their roots in the Civil Rights Movement, calling out racism as the number one mental health problem in the United States and challenging white social workers to get involved in responding to the problem head-on (National Association of Black Social Workers, 1968). Just four years after their establishment, NABSW took a stand on "transracial" adoption and unequivocally called for a moratorium on the practice of placing black children with white families for any reason (National Association of Black Social Workers, 1972). In their position paper on the issue, NABSW highlighted theories on child and identity development to support the proposition that placing a black child with a white family is not borne out of "altruistic humane concern for black children". Instead, they argued, "transracial" adoption was simply an expedient for white families who sought to expand their families through adoption in an environment where there were too few white children available. They argued that child welfare agencies should instead work to preserve black children in their families, preferring kinship care and, when necessary, building the resources of black foster and adoptive families. While the NABSW position on interracial adoption did not result in any actual ban on the practice, the frenzied debate on the issue brought attention to the issue of racial disproportionality in the child welfare system and helped focus efforts on family preservation and kinship care. More than 40 years later, the debate continues in peer-reviewed journal articles, newspapers, and online debates (Maillard, 2014).

As the child welfare system moved away from the institutionalization of children, the century-old tradition of removing Native American children into "Indian Schools" was terminated. Instead, new state-government-run child protection systems began to remove children from Native American communities and place them outside the tribe, often with white adoptive families. The Indian Adoption Project was a joint effort of the United States Children's Bureau, the Bureau of Indian Affairs, and the Child Welfare League of America (Palmiste, 2011). From 1958 to 1967, this federal program identified children, mostly living in poverty on tribal lands, and removed them from birth parents and families on the grounds of alleged neglect. These children were most often placed off tribal lands with white families. Nearly 400 Native American children were adopted during this time period into families in the Northeast, Midwest, and even to Puerto Rico. Contrary to the policies and practices at the time in traditional child welfare agencies, where white families were only allowed to adopt white children, these adoptions were deliberate governmental efforts to remove Native American children from their tribes, assimilate Native American children into "white culture", and purportedly offer them a "safer and happier life" (BBC, 2012).

Indian Adoption Project practices came under scrutiny around the same time that the NABSW took issue with transracial adoption. However, there was a clear policy response to the Indian Adoption Project. The Indian Child Welfare Act (ICWA) of 1978, which was discussed in Chapter 3, became national law.

Another national law systematized adoption policy and procedures across the United States. The Adoption Assistance and Child Welfare Act (AACWA) of 1980 was designed to respond to the growing number of children in out-of-home care who were freed for adoption but lacked a permanent placement for a number of years. The AACWA set out standards that aimed to preserve families where possible but moved quickly to adoption when preservation was not possible. While the aims of the AACWA were noteworthy and worthwhile, the changing political landscape in the 1980s along with social and economic challenges resulted in increased numbers of children in foster care and greater need for new, responsive policies.

After reaching a high of nearly half a million children in foster care in 1999, the number of children steadily decreased for more than a decade, to a low of 397,000 in 2012 (Child Trends Databank, 2018). However, the foster care population has increased by over 40,000 since 2012. This trend is largely attributed to the opioid epidemic (Radel et al., 2018). There were more than 437,000 children in foster care in 2016. As the number of children in foster care increases, so does the number of children in need of adoption. The number of children waiting to be adopted was nearly 102,000 children in 2012; in 2016 nearly 118,000 children were waiting for adoption (US DHHS, Administration for Children and Families, Administration on Children, Youth, and Families, 2017).

Key to successfully responding to current challenges is learning from the past. It is imperative that policymakers and practitioners understand the historical context for current adoption policy, so that past mistakes can be avoided in the present and in the future.

Different Kinds of Adoption

As previously noted, there are different kinds of adoption, although all adoption involves the same basic legal principle: replacement of legal parental rights and responsibilities. The focus of this textbook is on the child welfare system, with a significant focus on the child protection system. However, many adoptions in the United States take place outside that system in the sphere known as "private adoption".

Private Adoption

Private adoption can happen at any time in a child's life and, in some cases, even in adulthood. In practice, though, almost two-thirds of private adoptions happen in the first month of a child's life (Vandivere et al., 2009). Private adoptions, like adoptions from foster care, often involve placement with the child's relative. In fact, over 40% of private adoptions involve kinship placement (Vandivere et al., 2009).

Private adoption usually involves an adoption attorney or adoption agency, which serves as an intermediary between adoptive parent(s) and birth parent(s). Private adoptions require consensual termination of the rights of the birth parent(s). If the birth mother seeks to have the child adopted, any identifiable birth father must either provide consent or receive notification of his right to intervene before the adoption is finalized.

In private adoptions, the birth parent(s) get to choose the adoptive parent(s). When the birth parent(s) set their intention to place the child for adoption before the child is born, the birth parent(s) can work with an adoption agency to identify the chosen adoptive parent(s) at any time before the birth. However, the legal process to finalize the adoption cannot happen until after the child is born.

It is, obviously, illegal for birth parent(s) to sell a baby. However, all states allow adoptive parents to cover various expenses of the birth mother. Almost all states have laws that specify the type of expenses that can be paid by adoptive parents. Such categories include maternity-related medical and hospital costs, temporary living expenses, counseling fees, attorney/legal fees, and travel costs related to court appearances and accessing services. Some states provide that the reimbursement amount for expenses must be "reasonable". Some states have laws that clarify what adoptive parents are prohibited from paying birth mothers for. These categories generally include educational expenses, vehicles, vacations, and permanent housing (Child Welfare Information Gateway, 2017).

International/Intercountry Adoption

International or intercountry adoption involves American parents adopting children born in another country. While Americans have been adopting children from other countries since World War II, there has been a recent, steep decline in the number of children adopted from other countries. In 2004, nearly 23,000 children were adopted from outside the United States, with the largest groups of children coming from Russia and China. However, changing policies in various countries have resulted in restrictions on adoptions, either generally or specifically prohibiting adoptions by parents in the United States. China's shifting demographic policies have resulted in fewer adoptions, whereas concerns for ethical adoption practices have resulted in fewer adoptions of children from Guatemala and Russia. In 2016, just over 5,000 international adoptions were recorded, as compared to nearly 53,500 domestic adoptions (including adoptions from the child welfare system) in 2015 (Budiman & Lopez, 2017).

Single Parent Adoptions

In 2011, almost one-third of adoptions from foster care in the United State were completed by unmarried people. Nearly 90% of single parent adoptions from foster care were by single women. While laws do not discriminate against single parents in adoption, in practice single parents may face more obstacles to adoption than married couples. Case workers are tasked with identifying adoptive placements in the best interests of a child. In some cases, due to financial and other circumstances, a two-parent home may be preferred. However, there is growing recognition in the field that children can have great outcomes in single-parent families, especially with the right supportive structures in place (Child Welfare Information Gateway, 2013).

It is harder to adopt children internationally as a single parent. Not all countries allow single parents to adopt. In countries that do allow single parents to adopt, there might be different age or income requirements compared to married parents (Child Welfare Information Gateway, 2013).

While there are no restrictions on private domestic adoption by single parents, it is the least common way for single parents to adopt in the United States. Bias on the part of birth mothers and adoption service providers in favor of two-parent families is believed to be a significant reason for the low rate of single-parent, domestic, private adoptions (Child Welfare Information Gateway, 2013).

Adoptions by Same-Sex Partners

The United States Supreme Court decision *Obergefell v. Hodges* (2015) invalidated restrictions on same-sex marriage in all 50 states. The decision also had a series of repercussions on family law as it relates to same-sex parents. Married same-sex partners who intend to parent together can add both parents' names to a child's birth certificate at birth. Married same-sex partners can adopt non-biological children together as well. However, discrimination against same-sex partners is still not forbidden by law.

Private child welfare and adoption agencies continue to discriminate against same-sex couples. Non-married same-sex couples are not guaranteed the same rights as non-married opposite-sex couples, even by government entities. There are efforts in various forms of development seeking to ensure equal protection of all potential adoptive parents, regardless of their sexual orientation.

Second Parent Adoptions

Second parent adoption simply involves adoption of a child by a second parent. A second parent adoption allows a second parent to adopt a child without the "first parent" losing any parental rights. Second parent adoption can be used to allow children with one deceased parent to be legally adopted by a step-parent. Second parent adoption can also be used when a step-parent seeks to legally replace a birth parent who is not deceased. In these cases, the birth parent must either agree to relinquish their parental rights, or the parental rights must be terminated through the child protection system.

More recently, second parent adoption has been used to facilitate legal relationships between children and two parents in a non-marital, often same-sex, relationship. Second parent adoption for the purposes of facilitating the legal family relationship of non-married partners is not allowed in all states. In states where second parent adoption is not available, there are other legal mechanisms, such as custody law, that can allow both intended parents legal rights to a child. Additionally, there is a movement among states to allow for same-sex parents to be identified on a child's birth certificate. In these states, the need for second parent adoption for same-sex partners is greatly reduced.

Surrogacy vs. Adoption

With an increasing array of reproductive technologies available, there has been growth in the use of surrogacy. Surrogacy is the process through which a woman agrees to carry a pregnancy for another parent(s). Recent surrogacy practice involves a contract between the surrogate and the intended parent(s). The surrogate (or "gestational carrier") is impregnated with embryo(s) created from the genetic material of the intended parent(s). Whereas a birth mother cannot be required to relinquish her rights to adoptive parents after birth, a surrogate is not legally allowed to keep the child after birth.

"Open" Adoption

Open adoption is a form of adoption that allows birth parent(s) to continue contact with a child after relinquishing parental rights. Such contact is prescribed through a binding agreement between the birth parent(s) and the adoptive parents. There are various levels of "openness" in such adoptions. In some cases, birth parent(s) continue to have direct contact with the child throughout its life. In other cases, the birth parent(s) have contact with the child, but through letters or other forms of contact. Regardless of the level of "openness", parental rights and all of the privileges that come with those rights rest solely with the adoptive parents. While the birth parent(s) may establish a relationship with the child, decision-making is reserved for the adoptive parents (Child Welfare Information Gateway, n.d.).

Kincare/Kinship Adoption

Nearly a third of children in foster care are in the care of relatives (Generations United, 2016). When it is determined that a child will not be able to return to its parents, it is often preferred that they find a permanent placement, like adoption, with a fit and willing relative through kincare or kinship adoption. At least 25% of all states have laws that explicitly give preference to relatives in adoptions. Laws in some other states do not explicitly give preference to kincare adoptions, but the state may provide special support or incentives for such permanent placements over adoption by non-relatives (Generations United, 2018).

Kincare providers seeking to adopt are subject to state standards for the safety and well-being of the children. Standards for adoption may be more stringent than for foster care, but they also may be less stringent than those required of non-family resources. Once a child is adopted by the kinship provider, the kin becomes the child's legal parent, replacing the biological parent (Child Welfare Information Gateway, 2016).

Adoption from Foster Care

There were over 120,000 children in foster care on September 30, 2017, who were waiting to be adopted. Nearly 70,000 of them were already "freed" for adoption. There were nearly 60,000 adoptions from foster care in the previous year. Adoptions from foster care account for nearly one-quarter of all discharges from foster care in a given year (US DHHS,

Administration for Children and Families, Administration on Children, Youth and Families, 2018).

While the circumstances that result in a child being placed into foster care and subsequently adopted out of the child welfare system may be different than the situation that results in a child's adoption through the private domestic adoption system, the legal mechanisms required by both systems are similar in practice.

Adoption Practice

Legal Process of Adoption

Whether an adoption is coordinated through a private adoption agency or effectuated through the permanency plan for a child in substitute care (foster care) with a child protection agency, there is a specific legal process that applies in all 50 states, which involves the filing and approval of an adoption petition with a court.

In cases of international adoption, most of the legal adoption process occurs in the country where the child is born. American parents involved in the process of international adoption generally work with a US-based adoption agency, which coordinates the legal process in the child's birth country, as well as with the US Citizenship and Immigration Services here at home (Child Welfare Information Gateway, 2018). The remainder of the chapter focuses on the process of domestic adoption.

Availability for Adoption

A child must be "available for adoption" before an adoption petition can be processed. In private adoptions, the birth parents relinquish their parental rights at the time that the adoption petition is filed. In cases involving the child protection system, the state files a Termination of Parental Rights petition against the parents. The state must then prove by "clear and convincing evidence" that the legal severing of the parent-child relationship is in the best interests of the child (*Santosky v. Kramer*, 1982). Once this process is concluded, the child is "freed for adoption", and an adoption petition can be filed when adoptive resources have been identified and approved.

In cases outside the child protection system, birth parents need to consent to the relinquishment of their parental rights. If the birth mother is married to a man, her husband is assumed to be the father unless he claims and proves otherwise. If the birth mother is unmarried, but the father is known and involved, then he must relinquish his rights before an adoption can move forward. If the birth mother is unmarried, and the father is unknown or uninvolved, the adoptive parent(s) and the legal team processing the adoption should take care to make sure that every effort is made to identify the father and provide him notice of the intent for the adoption. While in most states an uninvolved father will not need to provide consent to adoption, there is always the risk that such a father will attempt to stop the adoption. In cases outside the child protection system, there is usually a short time period in which birth parents can change their minds about relinquishing their parental rights, generally around 30–45 days.

Identifying and Approving Adoptive Resources

In cases of private domestic adoption, adoptive resources or prospective adoptive parents may indicate their interest in adoption by applying to an adoption agency, advertising their willingness to adopt in the classified section of local newspapers, or publicizing their interest online. In cases of adoption from substitute care, prospective adoptive parents may already be serving as foster parents, or they may be exclusively identified as adoptive resources. Whether adopting from substitute care or through the private domestic adoption arena, all adoptive resources must submit to an adoption homestudy, which assesses their qualifications to parent.

The homestudy process varies by state and may differ depending on whether the adoption involves an adoption agency. Generally speaking, the homestudy process involves an orientation/education component, information gathering, and evaluation of the adoptive family's fitness to adopt (Child Welfare Information Gateway, 2015). When the adoption is taking place from substitute care, the child welfare agency is responsible for completing the adoption homestudy and presenting it to the court. In cases of private adoption, the evaluation of fitness is conducted either by the adoption agency or a privately hired professional, often a social worker, and presented to the court in a homestudy report. In all adoption cases, the judge has the final decision-making power regarding the fitness and appropriateness of the adoptive family.

Court Procedure for Adoption

Since so much is done to prepare a case for adoption before it comes to court, usually the court procedure is neither long nor too involved. The first step involves ensuring that all the appropriate persons receive notice of the adoptive family's intent to adopt the child(ren). While the rules regarding this process vary by state, generally, birth parents, other legal guardians, and, in some cases, adoptive children of a certain age need to be notified of the intent to adopt.

The second step involves filing the petition for adoption with the appropriate state court. In cases of private adoption, the attorney for the adoptive parent(s) will prepare and file the petition and represent the adoptive parent(s) in court. In cases of adoption from substitute care, the child welfare agency will prepare and file the petition and serve as the conduit for legal action throughout the proceeding. The petition generally contains identifying information for the adoptive parent(s) and child(ren); statements by the adoptive parent(s) expressing their willingness to adopt and their understanding of their rights and responsibilities; evidence of the termination of parental rights or the consent of the birth parent(s) for the adoption; and evidence that the adoptive parent(s) are fit for parenting (i.e., homestudy report).

The third and final step involves a court hearing on the petition. Although it is usually a simple formality, the process can be quite emotional. The judge asks the adoptive parent(s), on the record and under oath, if they understand the obligation they are undertaking by adopting the child(ren). The judge makes a decision whether the adoption is in the best interest(s) of the child(ren). If it is determined to be in the interest of the child(ren), the judge enters the adoption order and finalizes the adoption.

Social Work in Adoption Practice

In all forms of adoption, social workers are integral to the adoption process. Social workers can be employed by child welfare agencies, adoption agencies, and through private contracts with adoptive and birth parents. Social workers facilitate the process by recruiting and identifying adoptive resources; orienting birth and adoptive parents to the process; conducting adoption homestudies; and counseling birth and adoptive parents before, during, and after adoption.

Post-Adoption Realities and Concerns

Many people assume that once an adoption is finalized, that is the end of the story—everyone lives happily ever after. While that is the ideal scenario, it is rarely the reality. In the past few decades, various post-adoption policies and practices aimed at increasing the likelihood of adoption success have been developed.

Adoption Assistance/Subsidies

Ideally, every adoptable child in substitute care would be placed with a fit and willing adoptive resource who has no money concerns. However, that is not the reality for most American families, regardless of their willingness to adopt. When a child is in substitute care, their foster parent(s) receive financial and practical assistance from the state to help support that child. Many foster parents would be unable to adequately support foster children if the assistance was removed after adoption. Many adoptable children have medical and/or emotional conditions that require special attention, even after adoption. In recognition of the continued needs of children after adoption and the challenges faced by most American families, many adoptions from substitute care involve eligibility for post-adoption assistance and/or subsidies.

Adoption subsidies generally include some form of financial support. The type and amount of support varies by state and by circumstances. Some states may provide support only in cases of children with special needs or children who are "hard to place" (i.e., older children, children who have been in substitute care for an extended period of time, etc.). Other states may provide support for children without special needs. Some states may provide a one-time financial support at the time of adoption, while other states may provide ongoing monthly or annual financial support until the child reaches adulthood.

Adoption assistance can also include free health insurance, such as state-sponsored Medicaid; behavioral health support services; special equipment; and/or other support services (i.e., support groups, respite services, tutoring, etc.).

Loss and Grief

We usually associate loss and grief with death of a loved one. However, in cases of adoption, birth parents and adopted children may experience grief related to the loss of the familial relationship. Birth parents may experience loss and grief even before an adoption is finalized. Adopted children may not experience loss or grief until adolescence or adulthood. When and how these feelings are experienced are not universal. Therefore, responsive support should be tailored to meet individualized needs.

Identity

Identity is central to all people's development. Identity speaks to an understanding of who a person is and what their place is in the world (McGinnis et al., 2009). For adopted individuals, identity development may be more complex than for others. Adopted individuals' identities can include their birth family's experience, their adopted family's experience, as well as additional challenges, such as a lack of information or adoption stigma. Interracial/transracial adoptions may contribute further to challenges in identity formation.

Research findings support various practice and policy recommendations to increase opportunities for positive identity formation for adopted persons. Suggested practice improvements include initiatives to educate adoptive parents on how to support positive identity development in adopted children and efforts to reduce adoption stigma and stereotypes in the community (i.e., schools, media, etc.). Recommended policy developments include simplifying adopted persons' access to information related to birth families and supporting open adoption. For instance, a number of states have recently changed their laws to allow adopted persons access to their original birth certificates (Bergal, 2016).

Online Resources

- For more information on adoption: https://www.childwelfare.gov/topics/adoption
- Examples of the adoption petition form and other legal documents used in adoption can be found here: http://ww2.nycourts.gov/forms/surrogates/adoption.shtml

References

BBC. (2012). Native Americans Recall Era of Forced Adoptions. *BBC News*, November 21. Retrieved from: https://www.bbc.com/news/av/world-us-canada-20404764/native-americans-recall-era-of-forced-adoptions.

Bergal, J. (2016). With Push from Adoptees, States Open Access to Birth Records. *PEW Stateline*, August 12. Retrieved from: https://www.pewtrusts.org/en/research-and-analysis/blogs/stateline/2016/08/12/with-push-from-adoptees-states-open-access-to-birth-records.

Budiman, A. & Lopez, M.H. (2017). Amid Decline in International Adoptions to U.S., Boys Outnumber Girls for the First Time. *Fact Tank: News in the Numbers, Pew Research Center*, October 17. Retrieved from: https://www.pewresearch.org/fact-tank/2017/10/17/amid-decline-in-international-adoptions-to-u-s-boys-outnumber-girls-for-the-first-time.

CDC (Centers for Disease Control). (1999). Achievements in Public Health, 1900–1999: Healthier Mothers and Babies. *MMR Weekly*, 8 (38); 849–858.

Child Trends Databank. (2018). Foster Care. *Child Trends*. Retrieved from: https://www.childtrends.org/indicators/foster-care.

Child Welfare Information Gateway. (n.d.) *Open Adoption*. Washington, DC: US Department of Health and Human Services, Children's Bureau.

Child Welfare Information Gateway. (2013). *Adopting as a Single Parent*. Washington, DC: US Department of Health and Human Services, Children's Bureau.

Child Welfare Information Gateway. (2015). *The Adoption Home Study Process*. Washington, DC: US Department of Health and Human Services, Children's Bureau.

Child Welfare Information Gateway. (2016). *Kinship Caregivers and the Child Welfare System*. Washington, DC: US Department of Health and Human Services, Children's Bureau.

Child Welfare Information Gateway. (2017). *Regulation of Private Domestic Adoption Expenses*. Washington, DC: US Department of Health and Human Services, Children's Bureau.

Child Welfare Information Gateway. (2018). *State Recognition of Intercountry Adoptions Finalized Abroad*. Washington, DC: US Department of Health and Human Services, Children's Bureau.

Generations United. (2016). Children Thrive in Grandfamilies. *Grandfamilies.org*. Retrieved from: www.grandfamilies.org/Portals/016-Children-Thrive-in-Grandfamilies.pdf.

Generations United. (2018). Brief: Adoption and Guardianship for Children in Kinship Foster Care. *Grandfamilies.org*. Retrieved from: https://www.grandfamilies.org/Portals/0/Documents/2017/2018-Grandfamilies-Adoption-Guardianship-Brief%20(2).pdf.

Maillard, K. (2014). In Adoption, Does Race Matter? *New York Times*, February 2. Retrieved from: https://www.nytimes.com/roomfordebate/2014/02/02/in-adop tion-does-race-matter.

McGinnis, H., Livingston Smith, S., Ryan, S.D., & Howard, J.A. (2009). *Beyond Culture Camp: Promoting Healthy Identity Formulation in Adoption*. New York: Evan B. Donaldson Adoption Institute.

National Association of Black Social Workers. (1968). Position Statement. *NABSW—Harambee: 30 Years of Unity*. Retrieved from: https://cdn.ymaws.com/ www.nabsw.org/resource/collection/E1582D77-E4CD-4104-996A-D42D08F9 CA7D/NABSW_30_Years_of_Unity_-_Our_Roots_Position_Statement_1968.pdf.

National Association of Black Social Workers. (1972). Position Statement on Transracial Adoptions. *National Association of Black Social Workers*. Retrieved from: https://cdn.ymaws.com/www.nabsw.org/resource/collection/E1582D77-E4C D-4104-996A-D42D08F9CA7D/NABSW_Trans-Racial_Adoption_1972_Posi tion_(b).pdf.

Obergefell v. Hodges, 576 U.S. 644 (2015).

Palmiste, C. (2011). From the Indian Adoption Project to the Indian Child Welfare Act: The Resistance of Native American Communities. *Indigenous Policy Journal*, 22 (1), 1–10.

Radel, L., Baldwin, M., Crouse, G., Ghertner, R., & Waters, A. (2018). Substance Use, the Opioid Epidemic, and the Child Welfare System: Key Findings from a Mixed Methods Study. *ASPE Research Brief, Office of the Assistant Secretary for Planning and Evaluation, US Department of Health and Human Services*, March 7.

Santosky v. Kramer, 455 U.S. 745 (1982).

US DHHS, Administration for Children and Families, Administration on Children, Youth and Families. (2017). *AFCARS Report: Preliminary Estimates for FY2016*. Washington DC: US Department of Health and Human Services, Administration for Children and Families, Administration on Children, Youth and Families.

US DHHS, Administration for Children and Families, Administration on Children, Youth and Families. (2018). *AFCARS Report: Preliminary Estimates for FY2017*. Washington DC: US Department of Health and Human Services, Administration for Children and Families, Administration on Children, Youth and Families.

Vandivere, S., Malm, K., & Radel., K. (2009). *Adoption USA: A Chartbook Based on the 2007 National Survey of Adoptive Parents*. Washington, DC: US Department of Health and Human Services, Office of the Assistant Secretary for Planning and Evaluation. Retrieved from: http://aspe.hhs.gov/hsp/09/NSAP/chartbook.

15 Aging Out

What Does "Aging Out" Mean?

Most children placed in substitute care through the child protection system will be returned to their families. However, nearly 20,000 young people per year exit the foster care system simply due to their age (AFCARS, 2018). When a child in foster care turns 18 years old, they are an adult. As an adult, they have the right to live independently. However, many foster children lack the resources and supports that other children have when they turn 18. As a result, the child welfare system in all 50 states provides some level of service and support to adults as they "age out" of foster care.

Federal and state laws have attempted to respond to growing recognition of the unique needs of these foster youth. In 1999, the John H. Chafee Foster Care Independence Act was passed into federal law. It provided eligibility guidelines for youth receiving services to support the transition from foster care to independent living (as opposed to returning to their families or being adopted). The Act provided funding for services up until the foster youth turned 21. The specific content of programs was determined by individual states, but they generally included financial support for education and mentoring programs (Rosenberg & Abbott, 2019).

While there were programs prior to 2008 geared towards supporting some of the unique challenges this group faced, many states forced foster youth to officially exit the child welfare system either when they turned 18 or graduated from high school (whichever came last) (McCoy et al., 2008). The Fostering Connections to Success and Increasing Adoptions Act of 2008 (2008) was signed into federal law, and part of this child welfare law authorized the federal government to fund state-level child welfare systems to support foster children who need services after they turn 18. In order for a state to qualify for reimbursement for such services, the former foster child must meet certain disability, educational, vocational, and/or employment requirements. In other words, the federal government will not continue to provide funding for former foster children if they are not disabled, in school, or working. The Act specifically allows reimbursement for services until an individual turns 21 years old. When a person receiving support turns 21, the federal government no longer reimburses the state for any support or services for the former foster child.

In 2018, the Family First Prevention Services Act (Family First Act) amended the 1999 and 2008 laws to expand eligibility to all youth, ages 14 to 23, either in foster care or who had aged out of care. Prior to the Family First Act, states could focus programs only on those they deemed at risk. The recent change encourages states to provide services to help youth transition to independent living earlier, regardless of the decision to remain in foster care after 18 or not (Family First Prevention Services Act, 2018).

While all states provide some level of support to assist foster youth with the transition to independent living, the level and duration of support after the individual's 18th birthday varies by state. No matter what the level or duration of support provided, the now adult individual must consent to receiving the support.

Unique Experiences and Needs of Older Foster Youth

Older youth in foster care are different from younger children in foster care. The older a child is when they enter foster care, the longer they will stay (Rosenberg & Abbott, 2019). Older children enter foster care for different reasons than younger children. Older children are more likely to be victims of neglect, compared to younger children (Lee & Berrick, 2014). Older children are also more likely to have behavioral problems than younger children in foster care. As a result, older children in foster care have different needs than younger children. The child welfare system needs to be prepared to meet older children's distinct needs.

As all children transition from adolescence to adulthood, they experience various developmental milestones. Most of these milestones are related to changes in a young person's brain. As the brain matures in adolescence, young people explore their sense of identity. It is not uncommon for adolescents to act out behaviorally or respond emotionally when confronted with challenging personal situations. While these experiences are routine for all adolescents, youth in foster care are at a distinct disadvantage during this time. They are more likely to lack important resources that many of their peers undoubtedly, even if unwillingly, rely upon: parents and other family members.

As teenagers become more independent, they practice decision-making and adapt their coping skills. Youth often rely on family, teachers, and other supportive adults to help them in this time of transition. These important adults can serve as role models and mentors. They often provide guidance on emotional, educational, vocational, and financial decisions that will impact the youth's life for many years to come. Youth in foster care are more likely to lack access to supportive adults because they are more likely to be disconnected from family members, and their own parents might not be appropriate role models for healthy behaviors. As a result, foster care youth facing the transition to adulthood are at a major disadvantage compared to their peers.

Foster children are already known to experience more negative outcomes than children who are not exposed to the child welfare system. Unfortunately, foster youth who age out of the foster care system are similarly more likely to experience problems, especially compared to children who were never in foster care.

Young adults with experience in the foster care system are more likely to drop out of school before completing high school or college (Bersin et al., 2011), suffer serious mental health issues (including addiction) (Barczewski & Stout, 2012), be convicted of a crime (Courtney et al., 2010), experience unemployment and homelessness (Bender et al., 2015; Bersin et al., 2011), become parents at an early age (Courtney et al., 2010), and struggle financially (Courtney et al., 2010). It should come as no surprise that they are less likely to have health insurance or access needed medical care (Wilson-Simmons et al., 2016).

By age 26, approximately 80% of young people who aged out of foster care had earned at least a high school degree or GED, compared to 94% in the general population (Courtney et al., 2011). By age 26, 4% of youth who aged out of foster care had earned a four-year college degree, compared to 36% of youth in the general population (Courtney et al., 2011). Disproportionate educational attainment ultimately results in disproportionate employment opportunities, which can have lifelong negative consequences.

Children of color, specifically black, Hispanic, and Native American older children in foster care, are more likely to experience negative consequences than their white counterparts, likely because of the impact of continuing systemic and institutional racism. Older black youth in foster care have lower educational attainment than their white counterparts (Rosenberg & Abbott, 2019). Older Hispanic youth in foster care are less likely to remain in school, compared to their white counterparts (Rosenberg & Abbott, 2019). Native American youth who age out of foster care are less likely to be employed and, if employed, earn less than white youth who age out of foster care (Radel, 2008).

Since the turn of the twenty-first century, growing attention has been devoted to the unique experiences and needs of older youth in foster care and, specifically, those aging out of foster care into independent living. It has resulted in various state and federal policies aimed to meet these challenges head on. Research has shown that these efforts are worthwhile. The following section highlights some specific initiatives that have been found to positively impact outcomes for older youth in foster care and/or youth who have aged out of traditional foster care services.

Examples of Specialized Services for Foster Youth "Aging Out"

Extended Foster Care

While many youths in foster care would like very much to leave the child welfare system, research shows that choosing to remain in foster care after turning 18 has multiple benefits. Those who choose to remain in foster care after entering adulthood are more likely to complete high school, earn a college or vocational degree, and have a better job, compared to foster youth who choose to leave foster care earlier. Youth who choose to remain in foster care longer after entering adulthood are also less likely to become parents or be homeless. Why do these youth have better outcomes? Because while they are in "extended foster care", they receive services designed to help them develop independent living skills. These programs are largely funded through the federal legislation previously discussed in this chapter. These programs were not available more than 20 years ago. Thus, foster youth aging out of care today are likely to have better outcomes than those from an earlier generation (Rosenberg & Abbott, 2019).

Educational Support Services for Older Youth in Foster Care

After federal law was amended in 1999 and 2008 to allow state reimbursement for services for youth who remain in foster care after their 18th birthdays or services designed to support young adults recently discharged from foster care, state and local governments designed programs specifically tailored to meet the needs of their communities. The CUNY/ACS Fostering College Success Initiative (FCSI) in New York City is one such program.

Developed by the city of New York in 2016, the FCSI program provides support for youth in foster care beyond their 18th birthdays who are studying in an undergraduate program at the City University of New York (CUNY) and living in college dormitories. Eligible students have to apply and be accepted into the program. They can attend any of the 20 undergraduate CUNY colleges. Foster youth are provided with financial assistance, which pays for year-round housing in college dormitories; a daily stipend to cover essential items, such as phone, transportation, clothing, food, and books not already covered by financial aid or scholarships; and tuition support.

Also through the FCSI program, New York City's child protection agency, the Administration for Children's Services (ACS), partners with a local non-profit, New York Foundling, to provide college-based wraparound services. In addition, ACS's non-profit partner, New Yorkers For Children, provides back-to-school packages to all youth in the program. The range of supports offered through New York Foundling include help developing personal advocacy skills, navigating the complexities of being a college student, and accessing career development assistance through internships and professional opportunities. Students are individually matched with full-time academic tutors who support students with developing positive study habits, interacting with professors, writing college essays, and other academic skills.

The FCSI program was specifically designed in response to research from the past few decades that showed the negative educational and employment outcomes experienced by youth aging out of foster care. While preliminary results are encouraging, continued program evaluation will hopefully confirm that programs such as these have long-term benefits for these youth.

Mentoring Programs

Research shows that youth in foster care who have a strong, long-term relationship with one caring professional adult ultimately succeed at a higher rate (NYC Administration for Children's Services, 2016). Since many older youth in foster care are often at a disadvantage because they do not have secure attachments to traditional family, educational, and other community mentors, some state and local governments have developed mentoring programs to meet these deficits. One such example is a public-private partnership in New York City.

The Fostering College Success Mentoring Program (FCSMP) is a partnership between New York's Administration for Children's Services (ACS) and the giant financial firm, Goldman Sachs (Casey Family Programs, 2018). FCSMP was designed and implemented by Casey Family Programs, a national foundation focused on supporting improvements to foster care and child welfare. Students enrolled in the FCSI program, outlined above, are paired with Goldman Sachs employees who volunteer to be part of FCSMP program

Casey Family Programs designed the mentoring program to expose youth to professional and experiential opportunities through a series of one-on-one meetings and group workshops (Casey Family Programs, 2018). Students have the opportunity to become familiar with the Goldman Sachs corporate environment, learn about various employment sectors, and explore the roles and responsibilities of different jobs. Students also receive hands-on support with drafting resumes, writing cover letters, enhancing interview skills, and developing soft skills. They are invited to participate in an array of opportunities, including attending cultural events and workshops.

Goldman Sachs mentors must make a minimum one-year commitment with the opportunity to continue the relationship through graduation and beyond. Mentors make at least two contacts per month with their mentees (either by phone, FaceTime/Skype, or in-person), for a total of at least one hour of one-on-one mentoring during each contact.

Casey Family Programs will complete an evaluation of the FCSMP in the coming years. The goals are that the mentoring program will continue to show good outcomes for older youth in foster care and additional funding will be secured in a growing number of jurisdictions so that more impacted youth can benefit from the service.

Providing Resources to Professionals Who Support Foster Youth Aging Out

The previous programs explored in this section focus on services provided specifically to older youth in foster care or foster care alumni in young adulthood. Many social workers may be employed in other areas of practice but come in contact with older youth in foster care or foster care alumni in young adulthood. There are additional resources available to support social workers and other service providers who might have a higher likelihood of encountering clients who are in the process of "aging out" of foster care or who have recently left foster care. One such resource is the "Caseworker Resources" of the *Youth in Progress* website for New York State's Office of Child and Family Services (https://youthinprogress.org/index.cfm/ny-child-welfare-caseworker-resources/). This online resource has information for youth in care as well as for service providers working with adolescents in foster care throughout the state of New York. Resources include curriculum development, program design, and the statewide resource library catalog, which provides training, technical assistance, a lending resource library, and program development. While some of the resources are specific to New York State, others can be utilized by practitioners outside of state as well. Similar resource compilations may be available in your own state or local jurisdiction.

Online Resources

- Jim Casey Youth Opportunities Initiative of the Annie E. Casey Foundation: https://www.aecf.org/work/child-welfare/jim-casey-youth-opportunities-initiative
- Resources for Youth in Transition, Child Welfare Gateway: https://www.childwelfare.gov/topics/outofhome/independent/resources

References

AFCARS (Adoption and Foster Care Analysis and Reporting System). (2018). Preliminary FY 2017 Estimates, as of August 10, 2018: AFCARS Report, No. 25. *Administration for Children & Families*. Retrieved from: https://www.acf.hhs.gov/sites/default/files/cb/afcarsreport25.pdf.

Barczewski, J.M. & Stout, R.L. (2012). Substance Use Among Current and Former Foster Youth: A Systematic Review. *Children and Youth Services Review*, 34 (12), 2337–2344. doi:10.1016/j.childyouth.2012.08.011.

Bender, K., Yang, J., Ferguson, K., & Thompson, S. (2015). Experiences and Needs of Homeless Youth with a History of Foster Care. *Children and Youth Services Review*, 55, 222–231. doi:10.1016/j.childyouth.2015.06.007.

Bersin, S.C., Rhodes, A.M., & Curtis, M.A. (2011). Housing Experiences of Former Foster Youth: How Do They Fare in Comparison to Other Youth? *Children and Youth Services Review*, 33 (11), 2119–2126. doi:10.1016/j.childyouth.2011.06.018.

Casey Family Programs. (2018). Fostering College Success Mentoring Program: A Public-Private Partnership to Build a Better Tomorrow for Youth in Foster Care. *Casey Family Programs*, November. Retrieved from: https://caseyfamilypro-wp engine.netdna-ssl.com/media/1989_KM_Goldman-Sachs-NYC-ACS-report.pdf.

Courtney, M.E., Dworsky, A., Hook, J., Brown, A., Cary, C., Love, K., Vorhies, V., Lee, J.S., Raap, M., Cusick, G.R., Keller, T., Havlicek, J., Perez, A., Terao, S., & Bost. N. (2011). *Midwest Evaluation of the Adult Functioning of Former Foster Youth*. Chicago, IL: Chapin Hall at the University of Chicago. Retrieved from: https://www.chapinhall.org/research/midwest-evaluation-of-the-adult-functio ning-of-former-foster-youth.

Courtney, M.E., Dworsky, A., Lee, J., & Raap, M. (2010). *Midwest Evaluation of the Adult Functioning of Former Foster Youth: Outcomes at Age 23 and 24*. Chicago, IL: Chapin Hall at the University of Chicago.

Family First Prevention Services Act. (2018). Bipartisan Budget Act of 2018, Public Law 115–123, February 9.

Fostering Connections to Success and Increasing Adoptions Act of 2008. (2008). H.R. 6893/P.L. 110–351.

Lee, C. & Berrick, J.D. (2014). Experiences of Youth Who Transition to Adulthood Out of Care: Developing a Theoretical Framework. *Children and Youth Services Review*, 46, 78–84, doi:10/1016/j.childyouth.2014.08.005.

McCoy, H., McMillen, J.C., & Spitznagel, E.L. (2008). Older Youth Leaving the Foster Care System: Who, What, When, Where, and Why? *Children and Youth Services Review*, 30 (7), 735–745. doi:10.1016/j.childyouth.2007.12.003.

NYC Administration for Children's Services. (2016). Press Release: ACS and CUNY Announce Pioneer College Support Initiative for Foster Care Youth, November 2. *NYC: Official Website of the City of New York*. Retrieved from: https://www1.nyc.gov/site/acs/about/PressReleases/2016/jul15.page.

Radel, L. (2008). Coming of Age: Employment Outcomes for Youth Who Age Out of Foster Care Through Their Middle Twenties. *Urban Institute*. Retrieved from: https://www.urban.org/sites/default/files/publication/31216/1001174-Coming-of-Age-Employment-Outcomes-for-Youth-Who-Age-Out-of-Foster-Care-Through-Their-Middle-Twenties.PDF.

Rosenberg, R. & Abbott, S. (2019). Supporting Older Youth Beyond Age 18: Examining Data and Trends in Extended Foster Care. *Child Trends*, June 3. Retrieved from: https://www.childtrends.org/publications/supporting-older-youth-beyond-age-18-examining-data-and-trends-in-extended-foster-care.

Wilson-Simmons, R., Dworsky, A., Tongue, D., & Hulbutta, M. (2016). Fostering Health: The Affordable Care Act, Medicaid and Youth Transitioning from Foster Care. *National Center for Children in Poverty, Columbia University*. Retrieved from: http://nccp.org/publications/pdf/text_1165.pdf.

16 Ecological Perspective of Child Welfare

Families who are involved in the child welfare system commonly experience social problems. A multi-dimensional approach for assessing and working with children and families in the child welfare system looks at various factors that affect a family and can lead to child welfare involvement. Using a multi-dimensional framework like the person-in-environment perspective to understand and assess child maltreatment is an important consideration for child welfare workers and agencies. When child welfare workers fail to address external factors that affect the family's ability to care for children, child abuse is likely to continue. Using a model like the person-in-environment perspective allows child welfare workers to examine all systems impacting the family to create a case plan that addresses all of the child and family's needs, not just the immediate problem of maltreatment. Addressing all issues that might be impacting a child and family can lead to positive outcomes at the time of case closure.

Person-in-Environment Perspective

The person-in-environment perspective involves:

> the transactions between people and environments that, on the one hand, promote or inhibit growth, development, and the release of human potential and, on the other hand, promote or inhibit the capacity of environments to support the diversity of human potential.
>
> (Germain, 1981, p. 325)

When inputs or stimuli are insufficient, excessive, or missing altogether, an upset occurs in the adaptive balance, which is conceptualized as stress; the usual "fit" between person and environment has broken down.

(Germain, 1981, pp. 323–324)

Using a multi-dimensional framework to understand and assess child maltreatment is an important consideration for child welfare workers and agencies. The approach looks at a variety of factors that impact the child and parents. Frankel and Frankel (2006) indicate that models that focus on internal family dynamics fail to address external factors that affect the family's ability to care for children. Using a model like the person-in-environment perspective allows child welfare workers to examine all family systems and create a case plan that addresses all child and family needs, not just the immediate problem of maltreatment. Parents cannot parent effectively or without maltreating unless stressors from all systems are addressed. Addressing all issues that might be impacting a child and family can lead to positive outcomes at the time of case closure.

There are many factors to consider when using the person-in-environment perspective for assessment and intervention. Child and family well-being, mental health, addiction, housing, violence, and environmental factors all play a part in the functioning of the family and how much stress the family is experiencing. Examining each of these factors and implementing interventions to address each problem will decrease stress on the family and allow parents to focus on taking care of other issues, such as parenting ability. Typical factors to be assessed in a family and found in child welfare cases are discussed below.

Child and Family Well-Being

Family Status

African-American children are disproportionally overrepresented in the child welfare system (US Government Accountability Office, 2007). They are the subjects of a quarter of all instances of suspected maltreatment and a quarter of substantiated reports (US DHHS, Administration on Children, Youth, and Families, 2012). Additionally, about a quarter of the children in foster care are African American (US DHHS, Administration on Children, Youth, and Families, 2012). However, only 14% of children in the US population are African American (US Census Bureau, 2011). A study by Krase (2015) concluded that, nationally, educational personnel disproportionately report suspected maltreatment involving African-American children. The good news is that the percentage of black or African-American children in the foster care system decreased by 30% between 2008 and 2018 (AFCARS Report, 2019). In 2018, 44% of children in foster care were white, 23% were black or

African-American, 21% were Hispanic, and 11% were other races or multi-racial (AFCARS Report, 2019).

Poverty

The majority of child welfare cases in the United States involve neglect, and neglect is closely associated to poverty (US DHHS, 2008). Charlow (2001) found that, more often than not, child neglect is related to poverty, unlike other types of child maltreatment. Slack et al. (2004) indicate that certain aspects of poverty are more strongly related to physical neglect than other types of neglect.

Plotnik (2000) indicates there are several theories to support the relationship between poverty and maltreatment. The first theory is that low income creates parental stress, which can lead to higher chances of child abuse. The second theory is that parents living in poverty may be unable to provide adequate care while raising children. Additional factors related to the second theory include living in high-risk neighborhoods with unsafe or crowded housing and inadequate daycare. The third theory is that parental characteristics may increase the likelihood that parents are both poor and abusive. The last theory is that families living in poverty are reported to CPS more often due to greater scrutiny from community members (Plotnik, 2000).

Child–Parent Interaction

Families who abuse or neglect children seldom recognize the child's positive behaviors and react with harmful responses to the child's negative behaviors (Goldman et al., 2003). Goldman et al. (2003) found that parents who abuse or neglect "have been found to be less supportive, affectionate, playful, and responsive with their children than parents who do not abuse their children." Black, Heyman, and Smith Slep (2001) found that maltreating mothers were more likely to use harsh discipline strategies (e.g., hitting or prolonged isolation) and verbal aggression, while they were less likely to use positive parenting strategies (e.g., using time outs, reasoning, or recognizing and encouraging the child's successes).

Perry (2001) and Bolby (1988) discuss the importance of attachment and bonding between parent and child. If this does not occur, the child and the parent-child relationship will suffer. Perry (2001) confirmed early studies that babies and young children who are not touched or nurtured can lose the capacity to form healthy attachments. They can also experience physical and mental delays and problems. Factors that can affect bonding or attachment include child characteristics, the parent's behavior with the child, the environment, and the fit between the child's temperament and the parent's capabilities (Perry, 2001).

Communication

Connell-Carrick (2003) indicates that families who neglect have difficulty communicating and interacting appropriately. Many times, families who neglect are chaotic, lack emotional closeness, and are unwilling to take responsibility for their actions (Connell-Carrick, 2003).

Physical Health

Children with physical, cognitive, and emotional disabilities experience higher rates of maltreatment than other children (Crosse et al., n.d.; Sullivan & Knutson, 2000).

Mental Health

Parental Mental Health

It is not uncommon to see co-occurring substance issues and mental health issues in parents involved in CPS. Many researchers have found links between severe mental health issues and depression. Chalk and King (1998) indicated that severe mental disorders are not common even though some parents involved in CPS experience emotional or behavioral difficulties. Connell-Carrick (2003) stated that certain mental health problems with CPS-involved parents have been associated with child neglect. A study by Lee, Taylor, and Bellamy (2012) found that rates of parental depression were twice as high in families who were involved with CPS due to neglect. Burns et al. (2009) reported that in families involved with CPS, about half of the parents reported major depression. Mustillo, Dorsey, Conover, and Burns (2011) stated that "rates of parental depression in the child welfare population are elevated, even in comparison with other high-risk samples" (p. 165).

Infant and Child Mental Health

Between birth and the age of three, children are at the highest risk of maltreatment (Herrenkohl et al., 2008; Children's Bureau and NCANDS, 2010; US DHHS, Substance Abuse and Mental Health Services Administration, National Registry of Evidence-Based Programs and Practices, 2010). Children who experience stressful, traumatic events or household dysfunction have a higher chance of suffering developmental and health problems throughout their lives (Appleyard et al., 2005; Sameroff, 2000; SAMHSA, 2017). Short-term consequences of trauma can include externalized behavior problems; increased potential for depression, anxiety, and PTSD; difficulty with peer relationships; and cognitive problems (Herrenkohl & Herrenkohl, 2007; Herrenkohl et al., 2008; Margolin & Gordis, 2000;

Osofsky, 2003). Long-term consequences of trauma can include attachment issues. Children who are maltreated can have difficulty attaching to their parents or other caregivers (Herrenkohl et al., 2008), and as adults they may have difficulty forming intimate relationships (Perry, 2005). Additionally, some research has shown that children raised in stressful or maltreating homes tend to continue the cycle of violence in their own families as adults (Baer & Martinez 2006; Herrenkohl et al. 2008). Lastly, children who live in stressful or maltreating homes can experience physical issues as well. They may have a small head or build, and physical changes to the brain have been documented by researchers (National Scientific Council on the Developing Child, 2010; Perry, 2005).

Addiction

Children with parents who have addiction issues are more likely to face economic deprivation, family instability, poor parenting (Magura & Laudet, 1996), and domestic violence (VanDeMark et al., 2005). It has been estimated that the majority of child welfare cases, up to 80%, are related to parental substance abuse (Osterling & Austin, 2008; Young et al., 2007). Parental substance abuse has been identified as a factor in almost two-thirds of the out-of-home placements of children (US DHHS, 1999; Semidei et al., 2001). Chuang, Wells, Bellettiere, and Cross, (2013) indicated that the majority of parents' substance addiction treatment needs go unrecognized by child welfare workers. In addition, only about half of the parents involved with child welfare services who are referred to treatment actually receive services, and only about 13% complete treatment (Oliveros & Kaufman, 2011).

Housing and Homelessness

There is an association between housing difficulties and family involvement in the child welfare system. Unsafe housing or homelessness are two reasons why a parent might be charged with neglect. Housing disruption can make it difficult to keep families together, especially when many case plans indicate that parents need to have safe and stable housing (Courtney et al., 2004; Freisther et al., 2006; Pelton, 2008). Although child welfare workers and agencies are aware of family housing needs, there are often limited resources and funding available to assist (Shdaimah, 2008).

Violence

Interpersonal violence (IPV) is a significant concern in child welfare. Children exposed to IPV suffer short- and long-term effects, such as behavioral problems, anxiety, depression, low self-esteem, and aggression (English et al., 2009). Parent victims suffer physical and mental health effects (Nixon,

2009) and often find themselves in situations where they are unable to protect children from either viewing or being involved in the actual abuse (Nixon et al., 2013). Victims of IPV experience greater levels of stress (Levendosky & Graham-Bermann, 1998) and more difficulties in parenting, which can sometimes lead to maltreatment (Levendosky et al., 2006). Oftentimes, victim partners are charged with failure to protect a child from IPV or child maltreatment, and sometimes victims of violence lose custody of their children (Douglas & Walsh, 2010; Humphreys, 2010; Nixon, 2009). IPV batterers have been linked to child maltreatment (Gilbert et al., 2009; Hamby et al., 2010). Additionally, research indicates that child welfare workers have victim-blaming attitudes about IPV, they view victims mothers as being responsible for the abuse (Douglas & Walsh, 2010; Nixon, 2002), and they assume victims seek out violence by choosing the same type of partner for intimate relationships (Keeling & van Wormer, 2012).

Environmental/Community Factors

Social Supports

Families who have support networks tend to model positive parental behavior (DePanfilis, 2006). Support networks give parents access to alternative caregivers or provide additional support to the parent and the child. According to DePanfilis (2006), "Impoverished communities often lack positive informal and formal support systems for families." Quite a few studies have found that parents who maltreat children experience greater isolation, more loneliness, and less social support than non-maltreating parents (Blacker et al., 1999; Chan, 1994). Additionally, social isolation makes parents feel less emotionally supported and does not expose them to parenting role models (Harrington & Dubowitz, 1999). Researchers have not determined if social isolation is a contributing factor to child maltreatment or whether it is a consequence of maltreatment.

Neighborhood

Economically distressed areas have higher rates of maltreatment compared to other neighborhoods (Coulton et al., 2007). Ernst, Meyer, and DePanfilis (2004) suggest there is a relationship between unsafe or dangerous housing conditions and the adequacy of children's physical needs being met. Some of the relationship may also be due to the community acceptance of violence. Many low-income communities are associated with less social contact or support (Goldman et al., 2003). DePanfilis (2002) found that distressed neighborhoods include high levels of truancy, low academic achievement, high juvenile arrest rates, and high teen birth rates. She stated that when stressful living conditions continue over time, families are more likely to be reported to CPS for child neglect (DePanfilis, 2002).

Employment

Slack, Holl, McDaniel, Yoo, and Bolger (2004) found that employment had an inverse relationship to reports of physical neglect and that no difference existed between income groups for rates of fatal injury or emotional neglect.

Family Stress

Each of the areas discussed above have something in common. All can induce stress within the family system. Abuse and neglect risk increases when families experience stress. Lee, Taylor and Bellamy (2012) found that parenting stress relates to child neglect. DePanfilis (2006) indicated that neglectful families often experience financial difficulties, substance issues, illness, or housing problems, which makes coping difficult. Several studies have reported that neglectful families report more daily stress than non-neglectful families, and daily stress can worsen parent characteristics, such as hostility, anxiety, or depression (Goldman et al., 2003; Milner & Dopke, 1997). Researchers agree that CPS workers should look closely at stress. Classifying family stress using the following categories can assist the family and provide better interventions:

- Chronic environmental stress—background stress that is based in the environment and social structure, including dangerous housing, indigent neighborhoods, and chronic unemployment;
- Life events—stressful events and life transitions, including a job loss, the death of a loved one, or an eviction;
- Daily hassles—minor stresses that are present in day-to-day life, such as being stuck in traffic or problems at work;
- Role strain—stress caused by one's inability to fulfill a particular role. For example, a stay-at-home father may experience role strain due to mainstream society's expectation that fathers must always participate in the workforce.

(Tolan et al., 2004)

References

Appleyard, K., Egeland, B., van Dulmen, M., & Sroufe, L.A. (2005). When More is Not Better: The Role of Cumulative Risk Factors in Child Behavior Outcomes. *Journal of Child Psychology and Psychiatry*, 46 (3), 235–245.

Baer, J.C. & Martinez, C.D. (2006). Child Maltreatment and Insecure Attachment: A Meta-Analysis. *Journal of Reproductive and Infant Psychology*, 24 (3), 187–197.

Black, D.A., Heyman, R.E., & Smith Slep, A.M. (2001). Risk Factors for Child Physical Abuse. *Aggression and Violent Behavior*, 6, 121–188.

Blacker, D.M., Whitney, L.M., Morello, A., Reed, K., & Urquiza, J. (1999). *Depression, Distress and Social Isolation in Physical Abusive and Nonabusive Parents.* Paper presented at the American Professional Society on the Abuse of Children 7th Annual Colloquium, June, San Antonio, TX.

Bolby, J. (1988). *A Secure Base: Parent-Child Attachment and Healthy Human Development.* London: Routledge.

Burns, B.J., Mustillo, S.A., Farmer, E.M.Z., McCrae, J., Kolko, D.J., Libby, A.M., & Webb, M.B. (2009). Caregiver Depression, Mental Health Service Use, and Child Outcomes. In M.B. Webb, K. Dowd, B.J. Harden, J. Landsverk, & M. Testa (Eds.), *Child Welfare and Child Well-Being: New Perspectives from the National Survey of Child and Adolescent Well-Being,* 351–379. New York: Oxford University Press.

Chalk, R. & King, R.A. (Eds.). (1998). *Violence in Families: Assessing Prevention and Treatment Programs.* Washington, DC: National Academy Press.

Chan, Y.C. (1994). Parenting Stress and Social Support of Mothers Who Physically Abuse Their Children in Hong Kong. *Child Abuse and Neglect,* 18, 261–269.

Charlow, A. (2001). Race, Poverty, and Neglect. *William Mitchell Law Review,* 28 (2), 763–790.

Children's Bureau and NCANDS. (2010). *Child Maltreatment 2009.* Washington, DC: US Department of Health and Human Services, Administration for Children and Families, Administration on Children, Youth and Families, Children's Bureau. Retrieved from: http://www.acf.hhs.gov/programs/cb/stats_research/index.htm#can.

Chuang, E., Wells, R., Bellettiere, J., & Cross, T.P. (2013). Identifying the Substance Abuse Treatment Needs of Caregivers Involved with Child Welfare. *Journal of Substance Abuse Treatment,* 45 (1), 118–125.

Connell-Carrick, K. (2003). A Critical Review of the Empirical Literature: Identifying Correlates of Child Neglect. *Child and Adolescent Social Work Journal,* 20, 389–425.

Coulton, C.J., Crampton, D.S., Irwin, M., Spilsbury, J.C., & Korbin, J.E. (2007). How Neighborhoods Influence Child Maltreatment: A Review of the Literature and Alternate Pathways. *Child Abuse & Neglect,* 31, 1117–1142.

Courtney, M.E., McMurtry, S.L., & Zinn, A. (2004). Housing Problems Experienced by Recipients of Child Welfare Services. *Child Welfare,* 83, 509–528.

Crosse, S.B., Kaye, E., & Ratnofsky, A.C. (n.d.). *A Report on the Maltreatment of Children with Disabilities.* Washington, DC: Department of Health and Human Services, National Center on Child Abuse and Neglect.

DePanfilis, D. (2002). *Helping Families Prevent Neglect: Final Report.* Baltimore, MD: University of Maryland School of Social Work.

DePanfilis, D. (2006). *Child Neglect: A Guide for Prevention, Assessment, and Intervention.* Washington, DC: US Department of Health and Human Services Administration for Children and Families Administration on Children, Youth and Families Children's Bureau Office on Child Abuse and Neglect.

Douglas, H. & Walsh, T. (2010). Mothers, Domestic Violence, and Child Protection. *Violence Against Women,* 16 (5), 489–508.

English, D.J., Graham, J.C., Newton, R.R., Lewis, T.L., Thompson, R., Kotch, J.B., & Weisbart, C. (2009). At-Risk and Maltreated Children Exposed to Intimate Partner Aggression/Violence: What the Conflict Looks Like and Its Relationship to Child Outcomes. *Child Maltreatment,* 14 (2), 157–171.

Ernst, J., Meyer, M., & DePanfilis, D. (2004). Housing Characteristics and Adequacy of the Physical Care of Children: An Exploratory Analysis. *Child Welfare*, 83 (5), 437–452.

Frankel, H. & Frankel, S. (2006). Family Therapy, Family Practice, and Child and Family Poverty: Historical Perspectives and Recent Developments. *Journal of Family Social Work*, 10, 43–80.

Freisthler, B., Merritt, D.H., & LaScalla, E.A. (2006). Understanding the Ecology of Child Maltreatment: A Review of the Literature and Directions for Future Research. *Child Maltreatment*, 11, 263–280.

Germain, C.B. (1981). The Ecological Approach to People-Environment Transactions. *Social Casework: The Journal of Contemporary Social Work*, 62, 323–331.

Gilbert, R., Kemp, A., Thoburn, J., Sidebotham, P., Radford, L., Glaser, D., & MacMillan, H. (2009). Recognizing and Responding to Child Maltreatment. *The Lancet*, 373 (9658): 167–180.

Goldman, J., Salus, M.K., Wolcott, D., & Kennedy, K.Y. (2003). *A Coordinated Response to Child Abuse and Neglect: The Foundation for Practice*. Washington, DC: US Department of Health and Human Services, Administration for Children and Families Administration on Children, Youth and Families Children's Bureau, Office on Child Abuse and Neglect.

Hamby, S., Finkelhor, D., Turner, H., & Ormrod, R. (2010). The Overlap of Witnessing Partner Violence with Child Maltreatment and Other Victimizations in a Nationally Representative Survey of Youth. *Child Abuse & Neglect*, 34 (10), 734–741.

Harrington, D. & Dubowitz, H. (1999). Preventing Child Maltreatment. In R.L. Hampton (Ed.), *Family Violence: Prevention and Treatment*, 2nd edition, 122–147). Thousand Oaks, CA: Sage.

Herrenkohl, T.I. & Herrenkohl, R.C. (2007). Examining the Overlap and Prediction of Multiple Forms of Child Maltreatment, Stressors, and Socioeconomic Status: A Longitudinal Analysis of Youth Outcomes. *Journal of Family Violence*, 22, 553–562.

Herrenkohl, T.I., Sousa, C., Tajima, E.A., Herrenkohl, R.C., & Moylan, C. (2008). Intersection of Child Abuse and Children's Exposure to Domestic Violence. *Trauma, Violence, & Abuse*, 9 (2), 84–99.

Humphreys, C. (2010). Crossing the Great Divide: Response to Douglas and Walsh. *Violence Against Women*, 16 (5), 509–515.

Keeling, J. & van Wormer, K. (2012). Social Worker Interventions in Situations of Domestic Violence: What Can We Learn from Survivors' Personal Narratives? *British Journal of Social Work*, 42, 1354–1370.

Krase, K.S. (2015). Child Maltreatment Reporting by Educational Personnel: Implications for Racial Disproportionality in the Child Welfare System. *Children and Schools*, 37 (2), 89–99.

Lee, S.J., Taylor, C.A., & Bellamy, J.L. (2012). Parental Depression and Risk for Child Neglect in Father-Involved Families of Young Children. *Child Abuse and Neglect*, 36, 461–469.

Levendosky, A.A. & Graham-Bermann, S.A. (1998). The Moderating Effects of Parenting Stress on Children's Adjustment in Woman-Abusing Families. *Journal of Interpersonal Violence*, 13 (3), 383–397.

Levendosky, A.A., Leahy, K.L., Bogat, A., Davidson, W.S., & von Eye, A. (2006). Domestic Violence, Maternal Parenting, Maternal Mental Health, and Infant Externalizing Behavior. *Journal of Family Psychology*, 20 (4), 544–552.

Magura, S. & Laudet, A.B. (1996). Parental Substance Abuse and Child Maltreatment: Review and Implications for Intervention. *Children and Youth Services Review*, 18 (3), 193–220.

Margolin, G. & Gordis, E.B. (2000). The Effects of Family and Community Violence on Children. *Annual Review of Psychology*, 51, 445–479.

Milner, J.S. & Dopke, C. (1997). Child Physical Abuse: Review of Offender Characteristics. In D.A. Wolfe, R.J. McMahon, & R.D. Peters (Eds.), *Child Abuse: New Directions in Prevention and Treatment Across the Lifespan*, 27–53. Thousand Oaks, CA: Sage.

Mustillo, S.A., Dorsey, S., Conover, K., & Burns, B.J. (2011). Parental Depression and Child Outcomes: The Mediating Effects of Abuse and Neglect. *Journal of Marriage and Family*, 73, 164–180.

National Scientific Council on the Developing Child. (2010). Persistent Fear and Anxiety Can Affect Young Children's Learning and Development: Working Paper No. 9. *Center on the Developing Child: Harvard University*. Retrieved from: http://www.developingchild.net.

Nixon, K. (2002). Leave Him or Lose Them: The Child Protection Response to Woman Abuse. In L.M. Tutty & C. Goard (Eds.), *Reclaiming Self: Issues and Resources for Women Abused by Intimate Partners*, 64–80. Halifax, NS: Fernwood Publishing and RESOLVE.

Nixon, K. (2009). Intimate Partner Woman Abuse in Alberta's Child Protection Policy and the Impact on Abused Mothers and Their Children. *Currents: New Scholarship in the Human Services*, 8 (1), 1–17.

Nixon, K.L., Radtke, H.L., & Tutty, L.M. (2013). "Every day it takes a piece of you away": Experiences of Grief and Loss Among Abused Mothers Involved with Child Protective Services. *Journal of Public Child Welfare*, 7, 172–193.

Oliveros, A. & Kaufman, J. (2011). Addressing Substance Abuse Treatment Needs of Parents Involved with the Child Welfare System. *Child Welfare*, 90 (1), 25–41.

Osofsky, J.D. (2003). Prevalence of Children's Exposure to Domestic Violence and Child Maltreatment: Implications for Prevention and Intervention. *Clinical Child and Family Psychology Review*, 6 (3), 161–170.

Osterling, K.L. & Austin, M.J. (2008). Substance Abuse Interventions for Parents Involved in the Child Welfare System. *Journal of Evidence-Based Social Work*, 5 (1/2), 157–189.

Pelton, L. (2008). An Examination of the Reasons for Child Removal in Clark County, Nevada. *Children and Youth Services Review*, 30, 787–799.

Perry, B.D. (2001). Bonding and Attachment in Maltreated Children: Consequences of Emotional Neglect in Childhood. *Child Trauma Academy*. Retrieved February 8, 2018 from: https://childtrauma.org/wp-content/uploads/2014/01/Bonding-and-Attachment.pdf.

Perry, B.D. (2005). *Maltreatment and the Developing Child: How Early Childhood Experience Shapes Child and Culture*. The Inaugural Margaret McCain Lecture (abstracted), McCain Lecture Series, The Centre for Children and Families in the Justice System, London, ON.

Plotnik, R. (2000). Economic Security for Families with Children. In P.J. Pecora, J.K. Whittaker, A.N. Maluccio, & R.P. Barth (Eds.), *The Child Welfare Challenge: Policy, Practice, and Research*, 2nd edition, 103–104. New York: Routledge.

Sameroff, A.J. (2000). Dialectical Processes in Developmental Psychology. In A. Sameroff, M. Lewis, & S. Miller (Eds.), *Handbook of Developmental Psychopathology*, 2nd edition, 23–40. New York: Kluwer Academic/Plenum Publishers.

SAMHSA. (2017). Adverse Childhood Experiences. *SAMHSA: Substance Abuse and Mental Health Services Administration*. Retrieved from: https://www.samhsa.gov/capt/practicing-effective-prevention/prevention-behavioral-health/adverse-child hood-experiences.

Semidei, J., Radel, L.F., & Nolan, C. (2001). Substance Abuse and Child Welfare: Clear Linkages and Promising Responses. *Child Welfare*, 80 (2), 109–128.

Shdaimah, C.S. (2008). "CPS is not a housing agency"; Housing is a CPS Problem: Toward a Definition and Typology of Housing Problems in Child Welfare Cases. *Children and Youth Services Review*, 31, 211–218.

Slack, K., Holl, J.L., McDaniel, M., Yoo, J., & Bolger, K. (2004). Understanding the Risks of Child Neglect: An Exploration of Poverty and Parenting Characteristics, *Child Maltreatment*, 9 (4), 395–408.

Sullivan, P.M. & Knutson, J.F. (2000). Maltreatment and Disabilities: A Population-Based Epidemiological Study. *Child Abuse and Neglect*, 24 (10), 1257–1273.

Tolan, P.H., Sherrod, L.R., Gorman-Smith, D., & Henry, D.B. (2004). Building Protection, Support, and Opportunity for Inner-City Children and Youth and Their Families. In K.I. Maton, C.J. Schellenbach, B.J. Leadbeater, & A.L. Solarz (Eds.), *Investing in Children, Youth, Families, and Communities: Strengths-Based Research and Policy*, 193–211. Washington, DC: American Psychological Association.

US Census Bureau. (2011). *United States Census 2010*. Washington, DC: US Census Bureau.

US DHHS (US Department of Health and Human Services). (1999). *Blending Perspectives and Building Common Ground: A Report to Congress on Substance Abuse and Child Protection*. Washington, DC: US Government Printing Office.

US DHHS (US Department of Health and Human Services). (2008). *Child Maltreatment 2007*. Washington, DC: US Government Printing Office.

US DHHS, Administration on Children, Youth, and Families (US Department of Health and Human Services). (2012). *Child Maltreatment 2011*. Washington, DC: US Government Printing Office.

US DHHS, Substance Abuse and Mental Health Services Administration, National Registry of Evidence-Based Programs and Practices (US Department of Health and Human Services). (2010). Nurturing Parenting Programs. *SAMHSA: Substance Abuse and Mental Health Services Administration*. Accessed from: http://nrepp.samhsa.gov/ViewIntervention.aspx?id=171.

US Governmental Accountability Office. (2007). *African American Children in Foster Care: Additional HHS Assistance Needed to Help States Reduce the Proportion in Care (GAO-07-816)*. Washington, DC: US Governmental Accountability Office.

VanDeMark, N.R., Russell, L.A., O'Keefe, M., Finkelstein, N., Noether, C.D., & Gampel, J.C. (2005). Children of Mothers with Histories of Substance Abuse, Mental Illness, and Trauma. *Journal of Community Psychology*, 33, 445–459.

Young, N.K., Boles, S.M., & Otero, C. (2007). Parental Substance Use Disorders and Child Maltreatment: Overlap, Gaps, and Opportunities. *Child Maltreatment*, 12 (2), 137–149.

Index

Entries in **bold** denote tables; entries in *italics* denote figures.